RURAL AND APPALACHIAN
HEALTH

RURAL AND APPALACHIAN HEALTH

Edited by

ROBERT L. NOLAN, M.D., M.P.H., J.D.

Professor and Chairman
Division of Public Health and Preventive Medicine
Professor of Pediatrics
West Virginia University School of Medicine
Morgantown, West Virginia

and

JEROME L. SCHWARTZ, M.B.A., Dr.P.H.

Visiting Professor of Public Health and Preventive Medicine
West Virginia University School of Medicine
Morgantown, West Virginia

Professor of Community Health
University of California-Davis School of Medicine

With a Foreword by

Senator Edward M. Kennedy

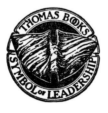

CHARLES C THOMAS • PUBLISHER
Springfield • Illinois • U.S.A.

Published and Distributed Throughout the World by
CHARLES C THOMAS • PUBLISHER
Bannerstone House
301-327 East Lawrence Avenue, Springfield, Illinois, U.S.A.

© *1973, by* CHARLES C THOMAS • PUBLISHER
ISBN 0-398-02605-X
Library of Congress Catalog Card Number: 72-87010

With THOMAS BOOKS *careful attention is given to all details of
manufacturing and design. It is the Publisher's desire to present books
that are satisfactory as to their physical qualities and artistic possibili-
ties and appropriate for their particular use.* THOMAS BOOKS *will
be true to those laws of quality that assure a good name and good will.*

Printed in the United States of America
N-1

CONTRIBUTORS

Garnett Bentley: Family Health Worker, Family Health Service, Elkins, West Virginia.

Robb Burlage, M.S.: Fellow, Institute for Policy Studies and Director, Appalachian Project, Morgantown, West Virginia.

Martha Ann Crider: President, Mountaineer Family Health Plan, Raleigh County, Beckley, West Virginia.

Abraham Drobny, M.D.: Chief, Department of Health Services, Pan American Health Organization, Washington, D.C.

Leslie Dunbar, Ph.D.: Executive Director, The Field Foundation, New York, New York.

Robert Eakin, B.S.: Project Director, Family Health Service and Administrator, Memorial General Hospital, Inc., Elkins, West Virginia.

Leslie A. Falk, M.D., D. Phil.: Professor and Chairman, Department of Family and Community Health, Meharry Medical College, Nashville, Tennessee.

William Taylor Fithian III: Fourth Year Medical Student, West Virginia University School of Medicine, Morgantown, West Virginia.

Charles B. Gilbert, D.D.S.: Practicing Dentist, Gilmer County, Glenville, West Virginia.

Doris Haddix: Family Health Worker, Family Health Service, Elkins, West Virginia.

David S. Hall, Ph.D.: Associate Professor of Sociology and Public Health and Preventive Medicine; Behavioral Scientist, West Virginia Regional Medical Program, West Virginia University, Morgantown, West Virginia.

Theodore P. Hipkens, B.S.: President, Appalachian Regional Hospitals, Inc., Lexington, Kentucky.

v

Murray B. Hunter, M.D.: Medical Director, Fairmont Clinic, Fairmont, West Virginia.

Gertrude Isaacs, Dr. Sc. Nsg.: Co-Director, Frontier Nursing Service, Hyden, Kentucky.

Helen L. Johnston B.A.: Rural Health Consultant, Community Health Service, U.S. Public Health Service, Washington, D.C.

Barbara Jones: Executive Director, Health Education Advisory Team Inc., Fairmont, West Virginia.

David H. Looff, M.D.: Associate Professor of Psychiatry, University of Kentucky College of Medicine, Lexington, Kentucky.

Frank W. McKee, M.D.: Dean, School of Medicine, West Virginia University, Morgantown, West Virginia.

William H. Miernyk, Ph.D.: Director, Regional Research Institute and Professor of Economics, West Virginia University, Morgantown, West Virginia.

Robert L. Nolan, M.D., J.D., M.P.H.: Professor and Chairman, Division of Public Health and Preventive Medicine and Professor of Pediatrics, School of Medicine, West Virginia University, Morgantown, West Virginia.

Leonard J. Pnakovich: President, District 31, United Mine Workers, Fairmont, West Virginia.

Milton I. Roemer, M.D., M.P.H.: Professor of Health Administration, School of Public Health, University of California, Los Angeles, California.

Jerome L. Schwartz, Dr.P.H.: Visiting Professor of Public Health and Preventive Medicine, School of Medicine, West Virginia University, Morgantown, West Virginia. (Professor of Community Health, School of Medicine, University of California—Davis.)

G. David Steinman, M.D.: Field Professor, Department of Community Medicine, University of Kentucky College of Medicine, and Daniel Boone Clinic, Harlan, Kentucky.

Joan White: Member, Board of Directors, Health Education Advisory Team Inc., Fairmont, West Virginia.

Eli Zivkovich: Special International Representative, United Mine Workers of America, District 31, Fairmont, West Virginia.

FOREWORD

In the spring of 1971, as Chairman of the Senate Health Subcommittee, I enjoyed the hospitality of the School of Medicine at Morgantown, West Virginia. During that visit, the Medical School's Division of Public Health and Preventive Medicine provided the Senate Health Subcommittee with invaluable background information and guidance through the counties surrounding Morgantown. That guidance, and the hearings which I conducted as Chairman of the Health Subcommittee in Kingwood, West Virginia, have indelibly impressed on the Subcommittee the need for reform in our nation's ability to provide health care to rural America.

The delivery of quality health care to Americans living in rural communities has become one of the most challenging and intransigent problems in our modern society. Social and economic changes in our nation during the last several decades have left many rural communities with little or no access to medical care, while at the same time leaving once prosperous rural farming and small mining and fishing industries unprofitable.

These changes have led to enormous human suffering and unrest. At their worst, they have resulted in entire counties where the average family income falls near or below the poverty line, whose health has deteriorated due to neglect, malnutrition and poor sanitation, and whose society breeds a despair seldom seen in the more fortunate areas of our nation.

On the several occasions when I have had the benefit of West Virginia's hospitality and instruction in the problems and the promise of Appalachia America, however, I have marvelled at the deep good will of rural Americans, and their persistent determination to make a good life for themselves in the country they know best.

It is therefore a special pleasure to foreword this volume re-

vii

sulting from a conference on Rural and Appalachian Health sponsored by the Medical School at Morgantown. The papers included here offer stimulating insights into both the nature of the problems of rural health delivery and the areas of promise. I share the hope of the contributors that the reader will be led by these papers to address his personal energies to the creation of a health care system which will provide rural America the best medicine our society has to offer.

EDWARD M. KENNEDY

PREFACE

T HIS BOOK IS a record of the papers presented at a conference at Mont Chateau, West Virginia, June 6-June 8, 1971, under the sponsorship of the Division of Public Health and Preventive Medicine, School of Medicine, West Virginia University.

Rural and Appalachian health problems and their solutions were selected as the theme because of the devastating effects such factors have upon people in these areas and family life there, the seriousness of the rural health problems in the United States and abroad, and their relative neglect by this affluent society. The editors, who served as conference chairmen, share a personal commitment to the favorable resolution of these problems. We believe the ideas recorded in this volume will make a significant contribution in that direction for some time to come.

Protocol often dictates that the composition of conferences be determined by rank and intramural politics. This can produce a dreary experience, emphasizing self-serving approbations without substance. Such considerations did not apply to this conference. We had the good fortune to enjoy the participation of a combination of scholars, health professionals, and those involved in rural health activities who could make the most effective contribution to this topic, irrespective of rank or station. Hence, it is neither surprising nor unanticipated that some of the views expressed by the contributors are simultaneously quite perceptive and controversial. With millions of rural Americans and other rural people throughout the world failing to share in the availability of health services, there ought to be far more controversy concerning rural health than this conference could generate. Inequality of opportunity in health and related matters demands a more adequate answer from a society claiming a commitment to equality.

We wish to acknowledge the freedom that we had to conduct the Conference and compile these contributions in book form.

The Conference was supported by a grant from the National Center for Health Services Research and Development, Department of Health, Education and Welfare. We enjoyed the encouragement and support of West Virginia University, particularly Provosts Charles E. Andrews, M.D., Ray Koppelman, Ph.D., and Ralph E. Nelson, Ph.D., and the assistance of Mr. William W. Reeves.

We also wish to express our acknowledgment to our colleagues of the Division of Public Health and Preventive Medicine, whose time and efforts so generously contributed both to the success of the conference and the publication of this book. We express special appreciation to Norene Thieme for helping to coordinate the conference; to Joyce Tapper and Janet Flynn for typing and editorial assistance; and to Lydia S. Aston, R.N., and Walter Morgan, M.D., for their interest and support. In addition, we would like to thank the individual contributors, who were of considerable assistance in facilitating the success of the conference and this volume.

ROBERT L. NOLAN
JEROME L. SCHWARTZ

INTRODUCTION

Over the century the United States has become increasingly urbanized in regard to concentration of population, resources, technology, and governmental and political activities. Most of our lives and interests relate primarily to the urban areas, although we still look to our rural areas for food and mineral products and recreation. Our involvement with rural America, however, has become largely impersonal. We seldom think of the origins of the fuel that provides our light, heat and air conditioning, until the specter of another coal mine disaster crushes out the lives of Appalachian fathers and sons and flashes briefly across the news screens. Nothing significant seems to happen until the next disaster strikes. Our awareness of the farm may not be revived until a severe drought or frost deprives us of some produce or raises prices in the city.

Approximately 27% of our people live in rural areas but 40% of the Nation's poverty is concentrated there. The rural poor in this country number some fourteen million; one out of four is poor in rural America. The President's National Advisory Commission on Rural Poverty reported in 1967: "Rural poverty is so widespread and so acute, as to be a national disgrace. . ." It is not surprising that poverty, dispersal of population, geographical inaccessibility, poor transportation, weak governmental and private institutions, and shortages of health manpower combine to deny so many of our rural countrymen and women access to health services. The implications of that deprivation are discussed in some of the papers in this book.

This volume consists of twelve original papers, a summary paper, and nine comments. All contributors are directly concerned with the health and economic aspects of rural America and most of them have made direct contributions to improving health care in Appalachia. In selecting the papers, we sought to achieve a balance between papers describing problems, those suggesting solutions and those detailing programs. Of the twelve original papers, four provide insight and background material on rural health problems; six pose solutions to those problems; and two papers describe health care models now being utilized in Appalachia.

The nine comments were contributed by a range of persons including a government rural health expert, a practicing dentist, a health administrator, an economist, two family health workers, and consumers representing labor, the poor and minority groups.

The book focuses first on the problems of rural areas. Toward this end there is initially an exposition of the attitudes rural Appalachians have toward health based on over 1,000 psychiatric interviews of Eastern Kentucky children gathered and evaluated by David Looff. His contribution is sprinkled generously with anecdotes from his extensive notes. He points out the barriers which make it difficult for outside agencies and professionals to reach Appalachian families. He describes the life style of mountaineer families which runs counter to the typical way agencies attempt to deliver health services. Looff provides suggestions for personalizing services to the rural poor, particularly mental health services, drawing upon the strengths of the Appalachian family.

The problems of rural America are summarized by Jerry Schwartz. His contribution is based on a study he made of rural counties in north-central West Virginia. The rural areas are described in terms of population decline, shifts in age distribution, economic activities and the extent of poverty. Schwartz outlines the available health resources and details the shortages of personnel and hospital beds and the paucity of public health programs. The major deterrents to attracting physicians lie with such factors as poverty, environmental problems, schools, and cultural and professional isolation.

William Miernyk summarizes the economic considerations and characteristics of Appalachia. He reviews the progress of the Appalachian Commission and discusses the strategy set by the Commission to concentrate on specific "growth points"—relatively large communities with growth potentials. This strategy is based on "economies of scale" and "external effects." He believes that economic development in Appalachia will occur largely in urban places and areas surrounding them. He discusses the notion of a regional health system and calls for a corps of mobile medical missionaries to provide services to the rural poor.

The major barriers to delivering health care are described by David Steinman from the viewpoint of the practicing physician. Distance from facilities, costs, and attitudes form the major barriers. Steinman presents the findings of several attitudinal studies of Appalachians toward health. He describes a program aimed at overcoming the barriers enumerated.

In a comprehensive paper, Milton Roemer highlights solutions to rural health problems attempted around the world. He points out that there is consistency between countries in problems of rural health and in solutions attempted. He describes efforts to increase manpower in rural areas through rural health centers and the reliance on regionalization. Roemer cites rural health care models from a wide variety of countries which have applications to rural America.

The role of the medical school in solving the problems of rural health is dealt with by Leslie Falk. He mentions six models of medical school participation in rural health and provides details of the Meharry Medical College's rural health experience. He emphasizes that the medical school and its teaching hospital must be the regional hub of the rural health care delivery system.

In a companion paper to Roemer's, Abraham Drobny draws on his experience in Latin America and suggests applications from our neighbors that could be used in our rural areas. He describes the use of assistant physicians in Venezuela to staff rural areas in Venezuela's regional health plan. Drobny also draws on the experience of other Latin countries in his proposals of solutions to our rural health problems.

Three authors have described the organization of health services and different methodologies utilized in rural settings to respond to health care needs. Murray Hunter reports the experience and impact of a multispecialty group practice serving a rural and semi-rural West Virginia mining area. He describes the relationship of a central group clinic and its branch clinic offices close to the homes of rural patients.

The development and approach of the Appalachian Regional Hospitals is presented by Theodore Hipkens. He describes the team delivery of rural health services via this chain of hospitals in Kentucky and West Virginia.

In the mountain country of Kentucky the use of the family nurse as a provider of primary health care has been the nucleus of the rural program of the Frontier Nursing Service since 1925. Gertrude Isaacs discusses the role of the family nurse in this rural setting, including the training, responsibilities, referral patterns, impact upon health manpower shortages, and other characteristics of this unique effort.

Leslie Dunbar has written a provocative discussion of our welfare system, its impact upon society as a whole and particularly upon the poor. He analyzes present national policy trends which influence welfare policy and offers some clear and precise recommendations for reform.

Valuable insights into the dilemma confronting the graduating medical student who is considering practice in an isolated rural county, is presented by Taylor Fithian. He discusses the necessary conditions of his own for such practice including those related to his family, the general community, the professional community and access to a major medical center, in a most forthright and perceptive manner.

Discussing the federal aspects of the rural health situation, Robert Nolan describes the present relationship between federal programs and rural health and then outlines the rationale for federal action. He offers an unusual combination of twenty-five specific recommendations for federal action to alleviate the conditions associated with unmet rural health needs in the United States.

David Hall's unique and perceptive summary and review merits special attention by the reader. The individual nine comments reflect the views and insights of a variety of rural people most highly qualified to speak first hand of the rural health problems from the depths of their own experience.

CONTENTS

RURAL AND APPALACHIAN HEALTH

Chapter 1

RURAL APPALACHIANS AND THEIR ATTITUDES TOWARD HEALTH

DAVID H. LOOFF

ULTIMATELY, in Appalachia as anywhere else, it is people that make the area important. It is the people of the southern mountains, in their region or in the places to which they migrate, who are the makers and carriers of their society and culture. They are the ones, primarily, who train the rising generation of their children and live their lives in either satisfyingly productive or bleakly nonproductive ways. Thus, although many agencies, bureaus, and departments of the Federal Government and the various state governments are rightfully concerned with natural resource development in Appalachia, with the building of new roads and schools, and with ways of fostering regional industrial growth, these concerns must not become the central ones. Rather, they must be viewed as they offer opportunities for people and as they affect the growth and development of children.

When we consider the difficulties of the people of Appalachia, whether in the mountains or in the cities, it is the manifold problems of the very poor that are the most vexing. The stable working class (although they are generally poor by federal income standards), the middle, and the upper classes in the region generally succeed remarkably well in providing for their health, education, and welfare needs. The most important developmental force accounting for this success is regional familism—close, interdependent family functioning, of which the most obvious expression is the extensive kinship system in the mountains. By ensuring that even limited resources will be shared among the extended family, particularly at times of crisis, familism stabilizes family life, structure, and functioning. This positive side of familism provides a steady state even for the very poor families. In this respect the

Appalachian very poor, unlike the often socially disorganized families raised in urban slums, possess a strength that can be tapped for redirection of their lives in many areas.[1] But one nevertheless encounters real problems in attempting to reach the Appalachian very poor with various health, education, and welfare service programs.

BARRIERS TO BE OVERCOME

At the present time, as well as in the past, any number of professionals from a variety of public and private health care, education, welfare, and vocational agencies have sought to bring their services to needy Appalachian people, whether these people be poor families who continue to live in the region or those who have migrated to urban ghettos. In their attempts to bring their expertise to bear on a particular area of a stricken family's life style, these outside professionals have frequently found apathy and resistance within the family itself. The sorely needed service or aid has not been accepted in any real sense of the term. More often the service, a welfare check, for example, has been silently taken and later, perhaps, not used for what appear to us as their greatest needs. Nothing really has been exchanged in the transaction except a sum generally inadequate to meet the family's needs for food, clothing, and shelter.

The paradigm holds true in the health care field. The living conditions of the very poor in Appalachia, their apathy, and the meagerness of resources have often forced medical care into inadequate, symptomatic, crisis-oriented patterns. Nothing has occurred in these encounters of failure (for that is what these abortive attempts to give and receive some sort of aid really are) because peoples' lives have not been touched. The helping professional feels rebuffed, unwanted, and unfulfilled as a helper. The potential recipient of the full measure of his aid, the Appalachian person in need, comes away from such an encounter feeling equally misunderstood and further rejected.

Thomas Ford points up several aspects of this barrier of resistance between the helping person and the family of the Appalachian lower class:

It is extremely difficult for "outside" agencies to reach these (Appalachian) families that most need their help. Community institutions, it has been noted, are not traditional mechanisms for handling "personal" problems in Appalachia. Numerous studies have documented that poor families do not participate much in community organizations of any type, including the church. And, because the personnel of these institutions are themselves often strangers, they frequently generate even greater insecurities on the part of those they are trying to serve. We have rather dramatic evidence of how traumatic a new experience can be to Appalachian children, especially when it must be faced apart from the family. The exaggerated fear of the unfamiliar institution is not confined to children. Stories abound of the very real apprehension and anxiety of adults forced by circumstances to utilize the services of an unfamiliar organization such as a hospital or a government agency office.[2]

The characteristic life style of the person in the Appalachian lower class, with its trained-in individualism, traditionalism, religious fatalism, action-orientation, and stoicism in manner and speech,[3] works toward an inner-directedness that cuts the person off from community institutions and from cooperative participation with a stranger in meeting, defining, and attempting to solve his problems.

This failure of many of our community institutions to reach the Appalachian poor was painfully demonstrated for me years ago in both the general health care and the mental health field. In the late 1950's, and again in the early 1960's, I was a trainee in a large university-based community-funded child psychiatry clinic in Baltimore and in Cincinnati. Both of these children's clinics were conducted in large hospital settings, and both ostensibly served, among others, families of the Appalachian migrant poor. My experience in both clinics sharply highlighted Ford's remarks. Migrant families were referred in great numbers to these agencies, but a majority of them did not return after meeting the large, strange staff in the unfamiliar setting and after encountering insistence on regular appointments for their succeeding visits. Too often, I feel now, these clinics, like many other community institutions that try to reach the Appalachian poor, took the position that their responsibility ended when the families had demonstrated low motivation for self-help by failing to return for care. Clinic services were available only on a take-it-or-leave-it basis. The customary rationalization of this position was that the clinics simply had insufficient staff to do otherwise. In one clinic, personnel were acutely aware of their failure to meet the needs of the Appalachian migrant poor, but were at a loss as to how to break through these barriers of apparent apathy or resistance.

The initial point at which these health care agencies failed in delivering health services to Appalachian migrant families was their lack of understanding of the life style of these families. The personal orientation of the mountaineer steeped in familism makes it very difficult, virtually impossible at first, for him to relate to total strangers in unfamiliar agency settings. In addition, his aversion to routines and to the agency's time-oriented casework schedules generally guarantees that he will not cooperate with the agency. This raises the question as to whether the particular life style of the person in the Appalachian lower class forever precludes his receiving help from various community institutions.

I think not, on the basis of my own sharply contrasting experiences in helping to deliver one type of health service to Appalachian families: field child psychiatry out-patient clinics in four local county health departments in eastern Kentucky. My earlier experiences, in Baltimore and Cincinnati, were ones of sharing many failures with my colleagues in the urban agencies. However, the experiences I have had in helping many families and their children through the Manchester Project, as our field clinics are called, over the past seven years have erased forever from my mind any doubts that all kinds of health services and, presumably, other types of services as well, can be brought effectively to Appalachian families. The essential difference between my experiences of clinical failure, on the one hand, and clinical success, on the other, is not, I feel, any factor that resides in me as a person or as a child psychiatrist. Rather, the essential difference that spelled relative success in the Manchester project was the different point of view of this work itself. It took squarely into account the fact that Appalachain people are person oriented; their characteristic of orientation to the self, to the intimate, and to the personal proved to be the point at which community agencies can begin to relate to them.

EXPERIENCE IN THE MANCHESTER PROJECT

It should be mentioned here that the Manchester Project was originally formulated by persons in the region, the county health officer and the staff of senior public health nurses, who were well acquainted with the families they served and, in turn, were accepted by these families as familiar givers of aid.[4] In a mountain area such a public health team is of much greater relative importance than its urban counterpart. In the first place, there are fewer doctors (in some counties, none at all). Besides, a high proportion of the patients are poor, from isolated parts of the area, and many of them would be unaware of the existence of medical and psychiatric care if they were not sought out by the nurses.

At the outset of our project, the local health officer and her nursing staff discussed local attitudes toward health care and some of their underlying causes. They pointed out that patients from mountain areas are almost overwhelmed by the scattered specialized facilities of the large hospitals and medical centers far from their homes. From time to time families have had to be referred to these centers for needed diagnostic and treatment services. These families were frightened, when away from their area and kin, by what they viewed as relatively impersonal institutionalized services. For these reasons, the nurses pointed out to us, Appalachian families tend to differ from the majority of Americans who want to and therefore can accept health care service wherever it is available.

The nurses gave us several compelling reason's why our jointly-staffed mental health field clinics for children should be based in the local health departments. First, there was the trend, already mentioned, for families to gravitate to the local health departments for their other health needs. Second, because of the traditional primacy of extended family or kinship ties, a family's acceptance of any health service depended upon their acceptance of the person who gave the service. Third, east Kentucky families shared certain other characteristics in their attitudes toward health care: they reacted to symptoms of disease and to the idea of disease itself with strong fears and anxieties. Many families, having little education and low income and hampered by barriers of language, were all too often confused, overly apprehensive, or even overwhelmed by health problems. Because of the traditional tendencies of the southern Appalachian individual to attempt to cope with anxiety by turning inward in his close family system, only a health care person long known and familiar could be accepted in a helping role.

The senior public health nurses understood this highly important familistic orientation. These nurses had flexibility in time and schedules, the mobility to reach people in isolated areas, and above all a visible proximity to the people who needed their services. In addition, their understanding of the culture equipped them for social encounter and interaction. Though themselves in the middle and professional class, the nurses were generally products of the cultural background of their people. They could therefore establish rapport with their people much more easily than could other middle-class professionals. Accordingly, the public health nurses, working through various health services, could counter or offset the traditional reluctance of many Appalachian families to seek help in problem-solving from outside agencies or clinics.

These points cannot be overstressed, so crucial are they, I feel, for the planning and delivery of all types of health services in the Appalachian region. In effect, many Appalachian families lack the psychological mobility that would lead them to seek specialized health care outside their local communities. They cooperate far better in extended health care if it is offered by familiar persons in familiar settings.

In our jointly planned and established work with emotionally troubled children and their families, we deliberately sought to use the diagnostic treatment services of the familiar and accepted public health nurses. We deliberately took our place with other public health programs in the region. In a sense, we rode for acceptance on the coattails of the nurses, who, long familiar to the families we served together, were called by their first names. When we would first meet with an understandably anxious new family that had been referred to one of our field clinics, we would frequently hear something like: "Faye came to see me Doctor. She said the teachers over at Lockard's Creek have been r'iled by Cindy. Faye brought me today. She says it's all right to talk to you." This was typical. The considerable extent to which we were able to win the trust and cooperation of individual patients and their families was due, first and foremost, to the nurses' understanding of the families we served together. They had, in advance, personalized our clinics. No family got service from a stranger.

The relative success of the Manchester Project in meeting many of the mental health needs of a substantial number of eastern Kentucky children (over 1,000 have been directly evaluated and treated, or provided consultation through teachers and other primary care-givers during the past seven years) and their families unquestionably demonstrated the effectiveness of planning for "personalization of services" for Appalachian families. Obviously, mental health services or even general health services are not the only kinds of services needed by these families. They have a host of inadequacies, calling for educational, welfare, vocational, and recreational services. The ultimate success or failure of the various agencies delivering these services to the Appalachian poor depends upon the extent to which each agency can personalize its approach. Jack Weller also underscores this central point, namely that the utilization of the personal approach is essential for agencies working with Appalachian families whose value systems stress the intimate and the personal.[5]

SUGGESTIONS FOR GENERAL HEALTH SERVICES

Just how this personalization of services is to be accomplished by various community agencies serving the Appalachian poor merits some discussion. First of all, the pronounced fear of illness shared by Appalachian families of all socioeconomic classes, based as it is on the threat to the family's solidarity, is one factor leading toward their acceptance of any health care service. It is certainly true that achieving better health for all family members is a crucial early step in the family's efforts to master the tasks confronting it.

The second consideration involves planning a health service regardless of the type, around familiar givers of aid in a familiar setting. If the service can be organized in this manner, it is more likely to reach the families it hopes to serve. For example, I feel that a healthy baby, prenatal, mental health, or other type of field clinic designed to meet the needs of the Appalachian migrant poor in a large city should be based in the migrant's community. We are well aware, from the work of several rural sociologists,[6] how Appalachian families migrate to and from little neighborhood pockets of their kinsmen and friends within large cities. It would be essential, then, for the planned health service to fit into this pattern—to locate within the migrant community in a building that is itself quite familiar to families in the area.

It would be equally essential for the health service to utilize as the prime givers of aid those persons to whom the families in the area naturally turn for talk and counsel. In eastern Kentucky, people have this relationship with the public health nurses in the local health departments. This might not be true in large urban settings, where the public health nurse may be just another outsider. If so, then a search must be made to discover just who it is that migrant families accept and relate to. It may be several of their number, generally women, who serve as informal but effective community leaders. These people should be employed as the ones who refer the families to the health service, convince them to come, and encourage them to continue. Their role in this work would be to bridge the emotional or resistance gap between the Appalachian families and the health care professionals. A prototype of such a person exists in the form of the home aides who are now functioning as bridges between the enrichment classrooms for very poor preschool children and their homes in ten eastern Kentucky counties.

One of these home aides, Mrs. G., whose family has lived for several generations in Owsley County, demonstrated for me several years ago just how effective a catalytic role such a local woman can play. A great yarn-spinner, Mrs. G. told me the story of one particular family she had helped. The C. family lived on a partially timbered hillside at the very end of their hollow. The wife, an extremely shy, reclusive woman of thirty-eight, seldom left the place. She spent her time tilling the garden, carrying water for cooking and washing from the creek, and attempting to keep up with the demands of her six wild children, who ranged in ages from four to twelve. Mr. C., forty-two, had worked for some years in the mines and drew a small pension for black-lung disability. This pension would have been adequate to feed and clothe his family, but Mr. C. shared with some of his men cronies in the area a strong liking for pedigreed coon hounds and for gambling. The money went in those directions instead of to the family. The children ran barefoot in all kinds of weather, were poorly fed and clothed, and consequently were frequently seen as sickly by the public health department. Mrs. C. never raised her voice in protest when Mr. C. bought the six rolls of half-inch, heavy-duty chicken wire for a new pen for his dogs, or bought another used car to make a trip to central Indiana to buy an expensive new coon dog. Mr. C. fed his dogs a well-balanced diet of fairly expensive dry meal, and he bought a new shotgun so that he could hunt with them. When not hunting or riding around with his cronies, he was gambling or cussing his kids who attended school only when they wanted to, which was infrequent.

Mr. C's behavior and lack of attention to the obvious needs of his wife and children had drawn down community anger and frustration upon him. School officials tried in vain to reason with him about his children's need for education and to impress upon him how he could help them by sending them to school regularly. Public health officials were appalled at the neglect of the children's health needs but their efforts to reach Mr. C. were likewise ineffectual. The public-assistance worker and a local minister had also talked with Mr. C. about his need to change his ways, again to no avail. Everyone in the community had given up on the man. "He's just stupid, and no count!" seemed to be the general feeling.

A year later, Mr. C's youngest boy reached the age of four and became eligible for the Owsley County day-care program. When the boy began to attend, Mrs. G. was assigned to the C. family as a home aide. She, like the other aides, had only general instructions to "go in there, see what the home's like, and do what you can to help."

As Mrs. G. told me later, her initial visits with the C. family were altogether different in approach from those of other community-agency workers. "I got up in that holler late one day after the longest walk. The car just wouldn't go any farther on that dry creek bed. I was thirsty, too, when I got there and Mrs. C. said she ain't got no fresh water yet; it's still down in the creek. But she didn't send no young'uns for it, and they was plenty of them running around, I tell you. Mr. C. just grinned and looked at me and said the only water he knew about up at the house was over in the dog's pen. Right then and there I see right off what shape things be in. I figger Mr. C. is stuck on them dogs and nuthin' else. So I decided to play it his way for a while. I said, 'I'd sure like to see them dogs,' and before another minute went by Mr. C. took me up to the pen. The two dogs he had were real pretty ones, especially the bitch from Indiana. I told him so—they were nice dogs. I like dogs as much as anybody, I guess, maybe more sometimes. And these were so friendly. I patted 'em, and Mr. C. was so pleased he let me open the pen and take 'em out. We walked 'em around until it was time for me to go. I told Mr. C. I'd be back to see him at the end of the week, and he grinned and said 'come any time!' He meant it, too, 'cause on Friday when I came back we took the dogs on a hunt in the woods—just Mr. C. and me. Plumb tuckered me, scramblin' over logs and in and out of swales, but I kinda liked it all, and Mr. C. sure did, I could tell that."

Three weeks apparently passed in a similar manner. On each of her twice-weekly home visits, Mrs. G. spoke initially only with Mr. C. and then spent her time entirely with him and his beloved dogs.

One day during the fourth week, as Mrs. G. related it to me, "We had a real gully-washer of a rain. I could see the dog pen saggin' all over the place and that-there soft dirt. Mr. C., he grinned and took me up there again. Made me mad—all that good chicken wire goin' to waste, saggin' down and fallin' down, and them pretty dogs havin' no decent place now. And I told Mr. C. so—I didn't care. I told him to fetch me a shovel, and he says, 'Miz Gibson, what you fixin' to do with it? You look mad enough to clobber me with it right off!' I told him I was mad all right, but I wasn't gonna hit him yet, if he helped me shovel out the new post holes to set that-there fence up right again. The idea, lettin' a thing like that go to rack and ruin! Makes a body mad! So we worked up there all afternoon. Tough it was and ever'time Ocie wanted to lay off and rest a spell I told him the next shovelful from me was for him. I told him it was a bald-faced shame to care for them pretty dogs so bad, that they had as much right as him or me to have a decent pen.

"The next time I come up there Ocie looked downright shame-faced if I ever did see a man look like that. He come up to me and he sez, 'Miz Gibson, you shamed me right. I guess I don't take care of nuthin' much.' Then Ocie told me he had sold the male dog to a neighbor and kept the bitch. He figured, he told me, that he wasn't doin' any better by his wife and the young'uns than with that dog pen, so he took the extra money he got and took them all to town for shoes and a picture show. And Mr. C. told me, 'Miz G., I'm gonna make us both proud,' and he did. I told him that any man who could shovel a post hole the way he done could go on the road gang (the OEO-funded Work Experience and Training Program) in the county, and he went." From that point on, there began to be evidence of better functioning in the C. family.

Mrs. G., unknowingly but in a natural, intuitive manner, had apparently followed the casework principle of helping a person overcome his adaptive weaknesses by working supportively with him from a position of his manifest strengths. Unlike Mrs. G., earlier community workers, in effect, had assailed Mr. C. for his weaknesses. This only increased his defensiveness and reinforced his indifference to his family's needs. Mrs. G., however, was genuinely fond of dogs, which gave her an immediate bond of rapport with Mr. C., whose dog care was his principal interest and strength at the moment. As a consequence of strengthening this bond by working with Mr. C. around his interests and supporting him in them, Mrs. Gibson found later that the man was receptive to her confrontation over his lapse of care. Ocie himself made the application to his family, when he felt genuinely liked and supported and was consequently less defensive.

Mrs. G.'s story is a very good basic demonstration of the effective way a local person can relate to poor families and assist them with a variety of tasks and problems. It is a person like her I have in mind as the bridge between various community programs and the people these programs are designed to serve. Further, the type of assistance rendered by Mrs. G. demonstrates again how effective frequent home visits are by the bridging person, both in leading to a clear understanding of a given family's weaknesses and strengths ("Right then and there I see right off what shape things be in") and in providing the most natural opportunities to work with others. These frequent home visits tend to reinforce the personal approach needed for a family's acceptance of a helper's suggestions or an agency's program. Visiting the home was a highly effective technique in the Manchester Project. Many times I have had the profoundly gratifying experience of finding my mental health recommendations better accepted on the family's front porch over a cup of their coffee than in my office across my desk.

SUGGESTIONS FOR MENTAL HEALTH SERVICES

Thus far, suggested outlines for the organization and the delivery of general health care services to the very poor Appalachian families have been drawn from our experience in the Manchester Project. These considerations are equally essential, I feel, to the conduct of local or even regional mental health-mental retardation services for Appalachian adults and children. I am suggesting, in effect, that our experience in the project can serve as a demonstration leading to the development of new mental health services for those living in rural Appalachia and for migrant families in the cities.

I feel that it is important to establish new mental health services for Appalachian children within already established general health clinics. Appalachian families are accustomed to gravitation to one setting for all their health needs. The setting itself, as well as the people who staff the agency, has grown familiar to them. In addition, there is much to recommend the inclusion of the home health aides in mental health work as well as general health work. The unique vantage point provided by their frequent home visits enables these aides to serve as monitors of the early development of the children in the families they serve. When they report on developmental lags and problems, early case intervention can be accomplished. You will remember that the Eastern Kentucky public health nurses, by checking frequently on the development of children in their districts, were in a prime position to help families redirect various features of the children's training if change were needed and to make early referrals to our mental health clinics if further evaluation and treatment were required.

Aside from these general considerations, common to both general health care and mental health services, two further factors, I feel, have important implications specifically for the mental health area. Both are drawn from our experience in the Manchester Project.

The first is that our project had a continual shortage of qualified psychiatric personnel. Even though the program was established, organized, and greatly extended by the public health nurses, we simply were not able to reach every family in the four eastern Kentucky counties that needed mental health services for their children. Knowing that this would undoubtedly be true as our work continued, we planned from the outset to extend our mental health reach even further by providing regular case consultations to the Head Start and day-care programs, to the schools, and to public-assistance and other agencies caring for children. The consultation program, which was a supplement to our direct therapeutic work with families, was designed to contribute to the effectiveness of these other community institutions that were seeking to help the people in other ways. For example, we, as consultants, attempted to help the staff of these agencies gain a better understanding of the several emotional stresses faced by people in the area who are very poor and some of the behavioral consequences of these severe and chronic stresses.

Sometimes, as a second point, we were able to point out the additional stresses which agency personnel themselves, however unwillingly, placed particularly on the very poor, and we discussed the need to eliminate these tensions before the workers could render their intended services. We sometimes encountered stress of this type resulting from the expression of overtly negative views toward members of the Appalachian lower class. Other agency workers sometimes held covertly negative attitudes that produced therapeutic apathy, rather than attitudes recognizing the potential for change in the lower class. Such attitudes, when continued, blocked the building of security and confidence, which must exist in order to establish and maintain a service relationship between the agency personnel and clients.

We felt that the negativism on the part of agency people, when it was found, was based on the familiar conflict over class identity known to sociologists and others who have studied various disadvantaged or minority groups. Those few agency staff members who reacted negatively to the poor in the region were reacting, I feel, to a threatened loss of their own hard-won middle-class, professional identity. At times they were made anxious by the public pronouncements of outsiders who threatened to blur class boundaries and to identify them with the Appalachian lower class. This accounted for the anger that many middle-class residents of the area felt toward Walter Cronkite's special broadcast, a CBS white paper on Appalachia released in 1963-1964, which seemed to them to deal solely with the local lower class. At other times, the middle-class professional person who attempted to assist a person of the lower class was made similarly frustrated and angry by what he felt was the poor person's calculated resistance to change. "I made it out of poverty, why can't he? He's just lazy and stupid!" was one way of expressing these attitudes. For other professional people, such direct angry acting-out of feelings toward those in the lower class was intolerable; these people instead internalized the anxiety-laden conflict based on class identity. The therapeutic apathy and nihilistic attitudes that subsequently developed prevented the effective working together of the helping person and his client. Our further role in the consultation program was to assist in identifying these feelings, if they existed, in members of agencies serving families in the area, and to attempt to bring the feelings out into the open for discussion and resolution.

APPALACHIAN FAMILY STRENGTHS

Two very important strengths that can be utilized by helping professionals to assist Appalachian children and adults are a marked capacity for essentially well-relatedness and an intense feeling-orientation possessed by Appalachian people in all socio-economic classes. Both of these strengths (some would call it parts of a person's ego functioning) are, I feel, derivatives of that marked focus on their children's infancy so characteristic of Appalachian families. I refer here to extensive data we obtained from a survey of Eastern Kentucky child development we undertook in 1964 prior to actual operation of the field clinics. At the time, we were looking for a normal developmental yardstick by which more appropriately to measure deviations from regional normative development in troubled clinic children.

We are well aware that one of the most important developmental tasks of the infant raised in any culture during the first year is to establish a satisfying dependency upon his mother. The mother-child relationship should be a close, satisfying, and supportive one. The previous work of other observers of Appalachian family life and our own survey on Eastern Kentucky child development suggest how abundantly true this is for local infants. Although in the years to follow Eastern Kentucky children encounter difficulties in development, particularly in children of the lower class, that first year or two of infancy is, from the infant's standpoint, relatively conflict-free.

Out of the mother-child relationship comes the foundation for the development of the child's feelings about himself, about people, and about the world in which he lives. If the relationship is a satisfying one, the infant begins to develop a sense of trust in himself and in his world, the first year being the decisive stage for the acquisition of this feeling.[8] He acquires a feeling of his own worth and adequacy and a feeling that the world is a pleasant, giving, and rewarding place. He begins to feel that people can be trusted. He is interested in the world. He investigates, explores, and tests. He attempts to communicate and to make meaningful interpersonal relationships. Relatedness, thus, is very much a positive derivative of an adequate infancy period.

Our first impression of this inherently strong capacity eastern Kentucky families of all three social classes have for trusting relationships was gained from their children. They related very well in clinic interviews, in their schools at the time of our consultation visits, and in their homes. Any initial reserve was soon dropped. Their capacity to relate led them to wait quietly, even with nonanxious anticipation, for their dental appointments in the health departments and for preschool physical examinations by unfamiliar visiting pediatricians. Most of us, as urban physicians, are accustomed to the waiting room crying and restlessness of young children. Thus, I was at first surprised to find eastern Kentucky children waiting quietly, without crying or excitedly giggling with each other. A passing adult could quickly relate with a waiting child and find pleasure in the encounter.

The eastern Kentucky child's capacity to form a quick, trusting relationship with the public health nurses and our medical team was a prime mover in the rapid progress many children made in treatment interviews. Success in nursing intervention, casework, and psychotherapy, including approaches in the general health field wherever it is practiced, depends on the relationship between therapist and child. It is the touchstone for any progress out of whatever difficulties the child may have. The same could equally be said of the parents of these children. Adults, too, related well with others, although the thawing out period was sometimes longer than the time required by the children. Once their initial reticence was overcome, however, parents made good use of the relationship aspects of treatment. In time, they were able to involve themselves in interviews with remarkable warmth and candor. Although many families were geographically and culturally outside the mainstream of county life, generally they related with us with no sense of personal isolation. In fact, their relatedness often combined such warmth, openness, and earthiness that we were reminded of the traditional spontaneity of young children. Gone were the layers of sophistication, telling the physician and others what families think should be said, that so often mark and impede initial treatment interviews with urban families. Such qualities of relatedness enabled the therapist to focus very quickly on family functioning.

Because so many of the families referred to the mental health clinic were action oriented, seeking primarily symptomatic relief for crises situations, the mutual capacity for relationship between the helping professional and parents had to be utilized quickly as the basis for helping a given family redirect its efforts with the children. Parents more readily tried out redirective suggestions made by the helping person because they had quickly established a bond with the outside person.

Of great interest to us as clinicians was the observation we made that the basic capacity for relatedness seemed to cross socio-economic class lines. For example, the often grubby, ragged children of the lower class we saw were frequently wild, impulse ridden, and manipulative. Yet, along with these traits was a warm way of reaching out to others that we interpreted as essential relatedness. It is striking how often the two personality traits, ability to relate well and yet simultaneously aggressive and wildly impulsive, find expression in all members of the same lower-class family.

Our conclusion from reviewing the developmental backgrounds of many children of the lower class in eastern Kentucky was that these children are well trained in basic relatedness from infancy on, but are not trained well in acquiring controls over their aggressive impulses. The children are well liked as babies and as older children, but in many areas they are allowed to do just as they please. Beyond the children's infancies, appropriate developmental lines involving a balance between gratification of needs and delays, limits, and controls are not readily maintained by lower-class families in eastern Kentucky. This seemed to account for the difficulties older lower-class children had with perceptual skills needed for orientation to a new environment, with communication skills, and with capacities to delay gratification and to establish internal impulse controls. During the infancy period itself, lower-class families as well as the others, freely gave of themselves to children. As an outgrowth of this, the children retained a considerable measure of the ability to relate with others in spite of difficulties with other capacities.

The implications for the mental health and general health fields of this capacity for relatedness should not be underestimated. All forms of health intervention (treatment) involve the giving and the taking of help in an interpersonal context. In my experience, and that of others, the relationship capacities of eastern Kentucky families are very real indeed, and these capacities are not dimmed by the families' migration to other settings. Presumably, then, those who work in any helping capacity with Southern Appalachian families, either locally or in another setting, will find mutual relationship a powerful working tool and thrust when Weller and others[9] refer to "personalization of services," they are talking primarily about this capacity for relatedness. After relationships are established, services of all types can then and only then be brought into focus.

The second consideration, that of the intense feeling-orientation of Southern Appalachian adults and children, is similarly a derivative from early child development in the region. Children are trained from infancy on to orient themselves to feelings rather than to words. This orientation to feelings is yet another aspect of the Appalachian person's action-orientation; "actions speak louder than words" and "a man is judged by his deeds, not his words" are but two ways of conceptualizing this orientation. Again, an orientation to feelings is a natural outgrowth of the Appalachian person's orientation to the intimate, the sensory, and the personal. In addition, what I call "regional nonverbality," a very important child development theme in the southern Appalachian region, is a powerful social reinforcer of this orientation to feelings rather than to language.

The use of language in eastern Kentucky presents some striking contrasts. On the one hand, there are clear indications that many people in the region find verbal communication very difficult. Theirs is an economy of language amounting to sparseness. The stereotype of the southern Appalachian mountaineer as a silent, taciturn individual is based on this difficulty. Neighbors of these people characterize them graphically as "quiet-turned." In our field clinics, we have followed a number of the silent members of these relatively silent families. The striking phenomenon is that the silent families exist side by side with others who are quite able to express feelings and ideas sensitively in words. The silent stereotype simply does not hold true for all.

The other impression we have gained is that difficulty in the use of spoken language, where it exists, crosses socioeconomic class lines. Though perhaps more individuals and families in the lower class and working class are notably taciturn, we have encountered many persons with similar difficulties in the middle-class group.

In addition to the silence of many individuals, other indicators show that nonverbality constitutes a training conflict in the Southern Appalachian region. Many eastern Kentucky families, particularly in the lower and working classes, set sparse speech models for their children. Such consistently presented training in silence is reinforced by consistent deficits in reading as well. Poor people, who are often illiterate or only marginally literate, not only cannot afford to buy magazines, newspapers, and books for themselves and their children but also have themselves been trained to place no real value on the written word. Accordingly, they have neither the means nor the inclination to read to their children. They do not generally encourage the children to read to them after formal schooling has begun. Where language is concerned, the training forces in many families amount almost to a vacuum.

The effects of this preschool verbal vacuum show up early. In the lower elementary grades, teachers are aware of the striking differences between the speaking children and the nonspeaking children, who are as well the readers and the nonreaders. There is evidence based on poor verbal scores made by many applicants taking general college admission tests and medical college admission tests that regional nonverbality affects many southern Appalachian adolescents and young adults as well.

Interestingly, these students who have language problems that impede their progress through reading and speaking in the academic curriculum from grade school on through college often come into their own in the more personalized aspects of their training. They frequently possess interpersonal skills to an exquisitely sensitive degree. Their early regional training in family closeness and relatedness mentioned before seems to pertain here. An outgrowth of this early training is their skill in observing and correctly interpreting the often-subtle, nonverbal behavior of people who are relatively silent. They have learned, in effect, to "follow the feelings" rather than the words. Thus, many of these students, in spite of marginal academic work resulting from their language problems, are able to find successful business and professional careers in fields requiring skill in personalizing services.

One must wonder how language disorders of this regional magnitude come about. I feel that at least four aspects of the functioning of the southern Appalachian family system deserve attention here. The first, raised initially by Thomas Ford, is that the family system is held together by norms of obligation and not necessarily by bonds of affection. Close, interdependent family ties involve training of the children in obligatory closeness; closeness frequently becomes a training end in itself. Situations that are viewed as potentially disruptive of close family ties are warded off. The existence of this trained-in feeling of obligation toward other family members, with an absence or at least an attenuation of ties based on affection, places a severe emotional strain upon individuals. This includes a sense of guilt. The person does not feel as he thinks he should toward other family members. This strain, Ford feels, may help to explain some of the intensive internal conflict as well as some of the striking lack of verbal communication inside families.

Presumably, then, the most severely strained families would show the greatest lack of verbal communication. We, and others, feel that this explains why families in the lower and working classes in southern Appalachia, the families having the greatest strains from many sources, have the greatest problems in using words as tools. As one impoverished mother put it: "I can't speak, when all my burdens sit so heavy on my chest." This would also explain, I feel, why the most socially isolated families frequently had children with emotional problems based on nonverbal themes. These children had fewer experiences with talking matters over with others than had their peers. Their social contacts had been largely limited on their own strained, silent families. Support of this view has come from the observations many have made regarding the spread of television into even lower-class homes. The children see and hear others speaking, even when family members cannot. Local teachers, for example, ascribe some improved verbal performance by lower-class children to the influence of television.

The second consideration about southern Appalachian family functioning that has implications for language training and language performance is closely related to the first. Perhaps it is simply a restatement of this first consideration. Child developmentalists have long been aware that a child's earliest training in speech functions occurs in an interpersonal context. Children begin talking, and continue to develop speech, by imitating the sounds and words of others. If those who train the child are relatively silent, the child has little to imitate except silence. Strained silence begets silence. In addition, strained-silent family members lack a most important tool for relationships with others, speech itself. With social contacts curtailed by silence, deficiencies which are frequently reinforced by educational and geographic isolation, older family members are often shy and socially withdrawn.

The third consideration involves dimension of southern Appalachian lower-class and working-class family functioning—the individual's and the family's orientation to action as opposed to the verbal consolidation, organization, and planning of one's experiences. This action orientation of the lower-class and the working-class southern Appalachian person is a logical outgrowth of the original mountaineer's rugged individualism and traditionalism.[9]

The fourth consideration is the considerable difference between the amount of language used by men and that used by women. Even in the eastern Kentucky middle class we have found women much more talkative than men. In consultations with teachers, for example, the women generally speak before the men do, and they speak longer. "Talk is women's work" was frequently heard, and heard across socioeconomic class lines. In many families this differential has had educational reinforcement. On the whole, the girls remain in school longer than the boys do. Action-oriented boys and adolescents of the lower and working classes eventually become bored with the word-oriented atmosphere of local schools. Many of them drop out. Later, the better-educated women, with further training in verbal skills, marry men who have far less formal schooling. We noted the frequency with which a middle-class eastern Kentucky woman with a completed high school or partial college education married a man who went no further than the fifth or sixth grade. In such family settings, men defer to their wives' better verbal skills.

Even in their traditional recreational pursuits of hunting and fishing in the mountains, men are trained from boyhood to "keep still." The silence of men engaged in these activities is an asset.

All these considerations overlap, certainly. But taken together, they have been a potent training force behind the language problems of many southern Appalachian children.

However, as I have indicated earlier, to emphasize training forces leading to language problems is to present only half the language picture. Nonverbal families in eastern Kentucky exist side-by-side with other families who are verbal. Our clinic work in the Manchester Project clearly indicates that many individuals and families, including some of the very poor, are able to express feelings and ideas sensitively in words. These verbal people have been exceptionally able to use word-oriented casework, nursing intervention, and psychotherapy.

Nevertheless, the importance of underscoring regional language problems where they exist in a particular family or individual is to point out the fact that the helping professional needs to learn to read the sensitive nonverbal, behavioral cues that silent Appalachian people give as evidence of the feelings they have, which they have not been able to present in words. Incumbent upon the helping professional, then, is the acquisition of the ability to follow feelings and to look for behavioral cues that exist.

Our experience in the Manchester Project related to this intense feeling-orientation of Appalachian families and their children, coupled with either regional language strengths or regional nonverbality, produces a consideration that is highly important to both the mental health and general health spheres. It has to do with the place of psychotherapy and social casework in the treatment of Appalachian families. Or, specifically, it concerns whether we have found that these verbal techniques have any merit in the treatment of the Appalachian poor.

I raise this point because at one time there existed in the nation the widely prevalent opinion that psychotherapy is neither the treatment of choice nor an effective treatment at all for very poor or even working-class people. Past failures of psychotherapy with some low-income groups in certain parts of the country, it is true, may have been largely due to the insistence on reconstructive, insight-oriented treatment of the kind long in use with the middle and upper classes. Several studies have documented the failure of such static forms of treatment to reach the poor.[10] However, our experience in Manchester Project clearly indicates that many poor Appalachian families are able to express feelings and ideas sensitively in words and therefore represent a group that can make effective use of insight-directed and even long-term psychotherapy and casework. These families exist side-by-side with other low-income, "nonverbal" families, for whom, I would agree, revised, action-oriented, crisis-model approaches seem more appropriate. Our conclusion is that the approach in mental health treatment must be flexible and fitted to the values, attitudes, and needs of the families being served.

CONCLUSION

It is obvious, I feel, that one cannot separate health from mental health and that both of these cannot be separated from social and cultural forces. In my recent book, *Appalachia's Children*,[11] I attempt to take a long look at regional child development themes in the southern Appalachian region, and at how these themes find expression both in the particular kinds of mental health problems children have in the area and in the particular strengths families and the children themselves possess. Finally, a section of the book focuses on some suggestions for redirecting the lives of young children in the area. In the book I tried to demonstrate the profound need for increased concern about what is happening to the rising generation—the children of eastern Kentucky, the children of the southern Appalachian region, and the children of the rural South. What kinds of persons are developing here, who are capable of realizing future opportunities that arise in their local or national setting? The implication of my work is that we must start at the beginning of the problem with the very young children. An attempt must be made to reach the problems of Appalachia where they start, in the fundamental child development patterns which close-in the individual in the lower class, particularly, and make it difficult for many to accept change.

As we do this we begin to see the critical importance of all types of community institutions in helping to shape the lives of these children. In urban, middle-class America it is the nuclear, or immediate, family that is of transcendent importance in the rearing of children; community institutions simply extend the family's training influence by reinforcing what is being taught at home. Today this pattern holds true for the southern Appalachian middle and upper classes. When we consider the southern Appalachian lower class, the very poor, and the poor yet stable working-class families, we face the problem of large gaps in family training of children. These training deficits create some of the particular kinds of problems affecting the children described in *Appalachia's Children*. I do not think we can expect southern Appalachian lower-class families, by themselves, to identify and remedy these training gaps. Instead, these families will need much continuing personal support from several kinds of community institutions. Many others feel as I do on this point. Thomas Ford not only has this same view but also suggests a broad outline for a community approach to this problem:

> It is my contention that the traditional family mechanisms have not been adequate to solve the problems of the poor in Appalachia or elsewhere in our modern society. Increasingly some of the burden must be shifted to other institutional systems. Before this can be done, however, the institutions must be able to reach the families, which thus far they often have not done very successfully. A two-pronged approach to the establishment of relations would appear to be in order. One approach would be to work directly with the families, helping them to function more adequately. The second approach would be to work with community institutions, aiding their personnel to gain a more sympathetic understanding of the lower class families they must serve. In my judgment, psychiatry has a great deal to offer to both approaches if we expand the psychiatric perspective of poverty to include not only the poor but also those who seek to assist them.[12]

In *Appalachia's Children* and this chapter I have discussed some ways of approaching those who present such vexing problems, and who do require outside assistance in order that their children may develop into individuals who can make choices and accept change. Call for help from those in the Appalachian lower class often must be painstakingly deciphered in the home and in the clinic before they can become the basis for positive, joint action. The rewards are profound. When progress begins, and we are relating to and working with a mountain man, his wife, and his children in this kind of joint endeavor, we see them beginning that extra ordinary experience which all people imbued with new hope undergo, namely, the flowering of their inherent capacity to grow and develop. The people of eastern Kentucky and of the southern Appalachian region have a remarkable and unique history. They have suffered long periods of struggle and despair. They have known economic and personal defeat. However, they also possess certain unique qualities. Many from the region have already utilized these strengths to build their own lives. Others, less fortunate, have yet to do so. Yet the strengths are there, too, waiting to be tapped and brought from a latent state into full activity. The mobilization of these qualities offers one of the great challenges to the health professions.

REFERENCES

1. Pavenstedt, Eleanor: "A Comparison of a Child-Rearing Environment of Upper-Lower and Very Low-Lower Class Families." *Am J Ortho-psychiatry, 35:*89-98, 1965.

2. Ford, Thomas: Discussion. Follows Looff, David: Psychiatric perspective on poverty. In *Poverty: New Interdisciplinary Perspectives.* Weaver, Thomas and Magid, Alvin (Eds.) San Francisco, Chandler Press, 1969.

3. Ford, Thomas: The passing of provincialism. In *The Southern Appalachian Region: A Survey.* Ford, Thomas (Ed.) : Lexington, Kentucky, University Press of Kentucky, 1962, pp. 9-34; Kephart, Horace: *Our Southern Highlanders.* New York, 1913; Campbell, John C.: *The Southern Highlander and His Homeland.* New York 1921; Odum, Howard: *Southern Regions of the United States.* Chapel Hill, North Carolina, 1936; Pearsall, Marion: *Little Smoky Ridge.* Tuscaloosa, Alabama, 1959; Chilman, Catherine S.: *Growing Up Poor.* U. S. Department of Health, Education, and Welfare, Welfare Administration Publication Number 13, May, 1966, p. 1.

4. Looff, David H.: Appalachian public health nursing: Mental health component in eastern Kentucky. *Community Ment Health J, 5, 4:* 295-303, 1969; Looff, David H.: Psychophysiologic and conversion reactions in children: Selective incidence in verbal and nonverbal families. *J Am Acad of Child Psychiat, 9, 2:*318-31, 1970.

5. Weller, Jack: *Yesterday's People: Life in Contemporary Appalachia.* Lexington, Kentucky, 1965, pp. 49-57.

6. Schwartzweller, Harry K. and Brown, James S.: Social class origin, rural-urban migration, and economic life changes: A case study. *Rural Sociology, 32, 1:*5-19, March 1965. See also Schwartzweller, Harry K. and Seggar, John F.: Kinship involvement: A factor in the adjustment of rural migrants. *J Marriage Family, 29, 4:*662-71, November, 1967.

7. Ford, Thomas, *op. cit.* [emphasis added] See also Johnson, Cyrus M., Coleman, A. Lee, and Clifford, William B.: *Mountain Families in Poverty.* University of Kentucky, Department of Sociology and Kentucky Agricultural Experiment Station, RS-29, 1967.

8. Erikson, Erik H.: Growth and crisis of the health personality. In *Problems of Infancy and Childhood.* Senn, Milton J. E. (Ed.) Supplement 2, New York, 1950.

9. Weller, Jack: *Yesterday's People.* Also helpful toward the concept of a "personalization of services" in a therapeutic sense in our work with eastern Kentucky families was Pearsall, Marion: *Little Smokey Ridge.* Tuscaloosa, Alabama, 1959.

10. Harrison, Saul I. and McDermott, John: Social class and mental illness in children. *Arch Gen Psychiat, 13:*411-17, 1965; Brill, Norman Q. and Storrow, Hugh A.: Social class and psychiatric treatment. *Arch Gen Psychiat, 3:*340-44, 1960; Overall, Betty and Aronson, Harriet: Expectations of psychotherapy in patients of lower socioeconomic class. *Am J Orthopsychiat, 33:*421-30, 1963.

11. Looff, David H.: *Appalachia's Children.* Lexington, Kentucky, University Press of Kentucky, 1971.

12. Ford, Thomas: *Op. cit.*

Chapter 2

RURAL HEALTH PROBLEMS OF ISOLATED APPALACHIAN COUNTIES

JEROME L. SCHWARTZ

I WOULD LIKE TO BEGIN with a selection from the opening of the thoughtful book by Rebecca Caudill, *My Appalachia.*

> My twin sister and I, so I have been told, were assisted on our arduous journey into life by a midwife, Usley Boggs. This event took place at Poor Fork, Kentucky, on a bitter cold night in early February. Three days later my sister died.
>
> My father hammered together a coffin of pine boards in which to bury my sister and covered it with black cambric. . . .
>
> My father laid my sister in the black-sheathed coffin, gently, as if he feared he might disturb her last, long sleep. Then he nailed the cover on the coffin, lifted the burden to his shoulder, and, bearing a much heavier burden within himself, set out across the Poor Fork River on the ice for the Sand Hill graveyard on the opposite side.
>
> Neighborhood men had already dug a grave—such a little grave!— in which to lay the coffin. Respectfully and silently they stood and watched my father lay his child in the grave. . . . No hymn was sung. No prayer was uttered. No word was spoken. Silence proclaimed the grief of my father and the warmth of the neighborly understanding that sustained him.
>
> Their duties finished, my father and his neighbors returned, each to his own home, leaving beneath the little mound not only the cold lifeless body of my sister but a part of my father as well.
>
> Once before my father had performed this sad rite. Twelve years earlier, when he and my mother lived at the head of Sand Lick, a son James, their firstborn, at the age of one and a half years had sickened and wasted away.
>
> In the crumbling old graveyards on the steep Appalachian mountainsides, the preponderance of little mounds, repeats the same story— no doctor, no hospital, no visiting nurse, no health services of any kind, not even a drugstore or a druggist. Only the few home remedies —quinine, castor oil, turpentine, and liniment—were to be found on the kitchen shelf, while in every neighborhood the old midwife went

29

her rounds with her baskets and her head full of notions about the birthing of babies.[1]

Although this description is that of a half century ago, even today many isolated communities have no doctor, no hospital, no visiting nurse, no health services of any kind; even the midwives are gone. What are the conditions in isolated rural counties—in terms of economic activity and health resources?

CHARACTERISTICS OF EIGHT RURAL COUNTIES

During the last year my colleagues of the Division of Public Health and Preventive Medicine of the West Virginia University School of Medicine and I have been studying conditions in rural counties. Specifically, we visited and interviewed a variety of persons in six rural counties in north-central West Virginia. I have also collected and analyzed economic, demographic, and health statistics relating to fifteen rural counties.

Some of the data for eight of these rural counties are summarized in Table 2-I to 2-III. I have selected these counties because they are isolated and contiguous. Of the eight, only two county seats are within one hour from a city of at least 25,000 in population and several county seats are over two hours from a city of this size. It should be pointed out that there are only eight cities in West Virginia of at least 25,000 population, and all but three are located on the state's borders. Only two cities in the state (Charleston and Huntington) have over 50,000 in population and none has over 75,000.

The eight counties chosen as a sampling of rural West Virginia consist of a land area of 3,200 square miles and a population of 81,000. The most populous county has 17,847 people and the least populated, 6,389. Density for the entire area is now twenty-five persons per square mile, down from thirty-six persons per square mile twenty years ago. The people living in these isolated counties are almost all white, there being only 0.6 per cent blacks.

None of the counties has an urbanized area and only one has an urban center of 7,300 population. The other counties are totally rural. The eight counties have nineteen towns, seven of them around one to two thousand people, but the other twelve are quite small (only two over 500 and six below 275).

TABLE 2-I
POPULATION CHARACTERISTICS OF EIGHT ISOLATED COUNTIES
OF WEST VIRGINIA

Population	Number	Change	Per Cent Change Over Decade
1940	128,028	+ 8,725	+ 7.3
1950	113,571	−14,457	−11.3
1960	94,369	−19,202	−16.9
1970	81,014	−13,355	−14.2

Urban/Town/County Distribution (Size)		1960	1970 Number	Per Cent Distribution	Per Cent Change 1960-1970
Total		94,369	81,014	100.0	−14.2
Urban	(over 2,500)	8,754	7,323	9.0	−16.3
Towns	(950 to 2,500)	18,178	17,052	21.1	− 6.2
Small towns	(100 to 949)	4,826	4,383	5.4	− 9.2
County		62,611	52,256	64.5	−16.5

Density	Persons Per Square Mile
1950	35.6
1960	29.5
1970	25.4

Extent of Poverty, 1966

Number of families	21,768
Number of poor families	7,694
Proportion of poor families	35.3 per cent

Sources: Bureau of the Census, U. S. Department of Commerce: *1970 Census of Population: Advance Report PC(VI)-50.* U. S. Department of Commerce, Dec., 1970.

Information Center, Office of Economic Opportunity: "Community Profile Project." Computer Printout, OEO, Charleston, W. Va., received December, 1970.

POPULATION LOSS

Three out of every four towns in these eight counties have lost population during the last decade—the loss is almost one-tenth in the large and small towns and one-sixth in the country areas. During the last twenty years the eight-county region has lost 29 per cent of its population. During the 1950's, the loss was 17 per cent, and during the 1960's, it was 14 per cent.

Table 2-II shows the changes in age groups for the eight counties. Despite higher death rates for older persons, there has been an increase in the proportion of the population over age 55. This suggests that older persons are returning to the rural areas.

TABLE 2-II
AGE DISTRIBUTION OF POPULATION IN EIGHT ISOLATED
COUNTIES OF WEST VIRGINIA

| | | 1970 | | |
Age Distribution	1960	Number	Per Cent Distribution	Per Cent Change 1960-1970
Totals	94,369	81,014	100.0	−14.2
Under 5	9,259	6,236	7.7	−32.6
5-14	20,314	15,515	19.2	−23.6
15-19	8,538	7,905	9.8	− 7.4
20-34	13,951	13,016	16.1	− 6.7
35-44	10,469	7,935	9.8	−24.2
45-54	10,857	9,033	11.1	−16.8
55-64	9,093	9,407	11.6	+ 3.5
65-74	7,139	7,103	8.8	− 0.5
75 and over	4,749	4,864	6.0	+ 2.4

Source: Personal calculations based on 1960 and 1970 census data.

This is supported by Photiadis' study of West Virginians who have moved to Cleveland and returned to Appalachia. He describes the returners as tending to be "older, unskilled, and with lower incomes and levels of living" than persons who remain in Cleveland.[2] When older persons are laid off from their jobs and cannot find employment or when they become sick or disabled, they return to their home county.

In contrast to the older age groups, there has been a population decline in just the last ten years in these eight counties for all other age groups, reaching almost one-fourth in the five to fourteen and thirty-five to forty-four year age groups and almost one-third in the under-five-year age group. (See Table 2-II) Another large loss occurs in the forty-five to fifty-four year group, down one-sixth. Age group losses have been even more drastic in some individual counties. For example, between 1960-1970 in Webster County the number of children under five declined 45 per cent, the five to fourteen year group was down 42 per cent and the fifteen to nineteen group was down 25 per cent. With an increase of older persons in this county, children under fifteen now make up 29 per cent of the population, whereas ten years ago they made up 37 per cent. At the opposite end of the age pyramid, persons fifty-five and over now compose 24 per cent of the population in contrast to 17 per cent a decade ago.

When one compares younger and older adults in West Virginia as a whole with adults in these rural counties, an older population is apparent in the isolated counties; in the state twenty to fifty-four-year-olds make up 41 per cent, while in the eight counties these groups make up 37 per cent of the population; on the other hand, the fifty-five and over group makes up 21.5 per cent statewide, but 26 per cent in the eight counties. The atypical population distribution in these rural counties has resulted in a substantially lower birth rate and a higher crude death rate as compared to the United States as a whole. In several counties the crude death rate exceeds the birth rate. Considering out-migration, we can understand why the population has declined so drastically. The out-migration of younger workers and able-bodied, middle-aged workers leaves behind an excessive proportion of the poor, the sick, the disabled, and the aged. Yet, the public services (welfare, health, mental health) are very weak and cannot handle this needy population. In addition, hospital and nursing home beds, physicians, dentists, nurses, and other medical resources are grossly inadequate to care for the people left behind and the elderly who have returned.

ECONOMIC ACTIVITY

Per capita income in 1965 ranged from 712 dollars to 1,449 dollars in the eight counties.[3] About one-fifth of the total personal income comes from transfer payments—welfare, veterans payments, and pensions. Unemployment for 1970 averaged over 10 per cent in four of these eight counties and two of them averaged 15 per cent unemployment for the year.[4] Although Professor Miernyk reports that conditions are improving in Appalachia,[5] this indicates that in the isolated rural counties economic conditions are not improving. As Miernyk states, "The economic progress that has been made in Appalachia has been largely limited to the region's urban counties. There have been few spillover benefits to rural, nonfarm counties."[6]

Very little new industry has been attracted to these rural counties despite concerted efforts by local groups in several of the counties. Instead, some small firms that were located in certain areas have closed down and gone out of business or moved away. The most workers are employed by the government (schools, city and county work, post offices), since manufacturing is limited in the eight-county area. Although the region contains enormous recoverable coal reserves, there is actually very little mining.

Only a small proportion of the work force is engaged in agriculture. Professor David Hall of West Virginia University presents the following account of farming in this area:

> Marginal farming still provides subsistence incomes for many families, with relatively little prospect for substantial economic growth and development. These farms mitigate against greater poverty and reduce migration to industrial areas where natives might increase their standards and level of living. However, the "outsider" who might spend a few days living with such a family would recognize as myth the notion that the rural resident lives a secure and untroubled life of rustic simplicity, supplementing his food supply by killing a deer from his front porch or picking wild berries.[7]

RURAL POVERTY

Typical of isolated areas, there is an overwhelming proportion of poor families in the eight-county region. Almost one-third of all families were classified as poor in 1966 by Social Security standards of income and family size.[8] Two of the counties had 44 and 47 per cent of their families below the poverty level. Only 3 per cent of all counties in the United States have a higher proportion of poor families than do these two counties.

Looking at all of Appalachia or at the entire state, without separating out urban areas from the rural ones or mountain and isolated sections from rural farm areas, is a misleading approach. In 1966, for example, West Virginia had 23 per cent of its families classified as poor, but each of these eight counties has a higher proportion of poverty families than does the state as a whole and the two counties referred to previously have twice as many poor families as does the state.[9]

Welfare payments are quite low, and there even appear to be wide differences among payments to recipients within the eight-county region. Average monthly payments for Aid to Families with Dependent Children is about 90 dollars. Only a small proportion of the poverty families are on welfare as most of the poor families belong to the working poor—wage earners at minimal salaries. Rural poverty is often typified by crowded living conditions, poor housing, inadequate sewage disposal, insufficient clothing, and nutritional deficiencies. The rural poor lack the resources to pay for health care and their resulting disabilities increase their dependence. Milton Roemer[10] and Dave Steinman[11] describe other special health needs and characteristics of the rural poor. One critical barrier to the receipt of health care, particularly by people who qualify for Medicaid or Medicare, is the lack of transportation to places where there are doctors and hospitals.

HEALTH RESOURCES

Throughout the region there is a shortage of health practitioners, and the few practicing physicians and dentists are overworked. Physicians practicing alone can find no relief and report that people are resentful if they leave town for even one afternoon or evening.

Table 2-III shows the distribution of health personnel. There are only 23 physicians and seven dentists in active practice in the eight-county area. Two of the counties, Clay and Doddridge, have neither a physician nor a dentist. In 1968, Doddridge County built a modern medical clinic with local resources. Three different physicians have covered the county for nineteen out of the last forty-two months. Two of the physicians were foreign-trained, one from Thailand and one from the Philippines. The last physician was a qualified surgeon who was well-liked; however, he left when he could not secure a permanent license. Since December, 1969, the building has remained empty and the county has been without a physician. Clay, the other county, with a population of 9,300, has offered a guarantee of 36,000 dollars to a physician, 24,000 dollars to a dentist, and 18,000 dollars to a pharmacist if any of these professionals will agree to practice in the county. The Clay County Clerk reports that only a few physicians have been interviewed for the position.[12] Clay has been without a doctor since June of 1970 when their only doctor retired.

TABLE 2-III

HEALTH PROFESSIONALS PRACTICING IN EIGHT ISOLATED
COUNTIES OF WEST VIRGINIA

	Number	Population Ratios	Eight-County Area per 100,000*	West Virginia per 100,000*
Physicians and Osteopaths	23	1/ 3,522	28.4	91.7 (1968-69)
Dentists	7	1/11,573	8.6	36.1 (1967)
Nurses RN	82	1/ 988	101.2	276.6 (1966)
Pharmacists	20	1/ 4,051	24.7	29.1 (1968)
LPN's	73	1/ 1,110		
Physical therapists	0	—		
Medical technicians	6	1/13,502		
Emergency Services—Transportation				
Local hospital	0			
Rescue squad	0			
Ambulance service	1			
Fire or police department	1			
Funeral homes	19			
Other	0			
Public Health Personnel, September 1969				
Nurses	9	1/ 9,001	11.1	
Sanitarians	3	1/27,004	3.7	
Clerks	9	1/ 9,001		
Home health aides	1	1/81,014		

Sources: Regional Medical Program, West Virginia University Medical Center: Data
Summary Sheet, 1969.
West Virginia Department of Health Personnel Directory, September, 1969.
Telephone survey, September, 1970.

*U:S. ratios per 100,000: Active non-federal dentists (1968) —47; active non-federal
physicians (1967) —130; practicing RN's (1969) —338; pharmacists (1969) —63.
(Source: National Center for Health Statistics: *Health Resources Statistics,* 1969.)

In 1938 when this eight-county area had 126,000 people, there were at least five doctors in each county—as many as fifteen physicians in three of the counties. Clay County, referred to before, had five physicians, and Doddridge, which has none today, had ten in practice. Population ratios for these eight counties show eighty physicians per 100,000 persons in 1938, sixty-five in 1950, fifty-three in 1960, and twenty-eight today.[13] This compares to ninety-two physicians per 100,000 for the state of West Virginia as a whole.

These isolated counties have never had many dentists, and as the old dentists die off, few are replaced. In 1958 there were twenty-four dentists in the eight counties, which is more than three times as many as are practicing today in this region. The lack of dental care is one of the most critical health problems of rural people. Interviews of rural residents in one county revealed that over the period of one year less than one-quarter of the families had any member visit a dentist.

Four of the eight counties have hospitals. The counties without hospitals have great difficulty in recruiting young physicians because there are no colleagues to work with or facilities. Outside of funeral vans, emergency vehicles are available in only two of the counties. There are no physical therapists in the entire region and there are only six medical technicians. Even though these areas have many aged persons, there is almost a total lack of skilled nursing care, home health services, rehabilitative care, and extended health care. Family planning services are also generally lacking in rural areas although our own Family Planning Project has initiated services in some of these isolated communities.

Public health programs are very narrow and limited in these rural areas. Minimal public health services should include some attention to environmental hazards and sanitation; clinicals for prenatal care; vaccinations; healthy child care; home visits to new mothers, the disabled, and the aged; health education on such subjects as safety, nutrition, hygiene, and cigarette smoking; and some screening of school children for eye, dental, and serious health problems. As noted in Table 2-III, the staffs of rural health departments are minimal: sanitarians in only three of the eight counties, only one home health aide, and just nine nurses in the entire area.* Generally, the only functions of the local part-time health officer are to sign official papers, attend meetings,

---

*It should be noted that Clay County is receiving services of staff supplied by the State Health Department. Two pediatricians hold clinics in Clay twice per week; nurses, dentists, dental hygienists, nutritionists, and laboratory technicians also come from Charleston on a regular basis.

and make himself available for telephone consultation. One county health officer told us he rarely goes to the health department.

The following is a description of health resources in Gilmer County. Glenville, the county seat, is the home of two osteopaths, two general practitioners, and one dentist. However, the two general practitioners are both over eighty years of age and in poor health; the two osteopaths, both nearly sixty years and aged beyond their years, have exceedingly busy practices. One of them fills in as the physician for Glenville State College since the College has been unable to recruit its own doctor. The dental resident in Glenville is young and conscientious; he handles virtually all the dentistry for Gilmer, as well as caring for residents from neighboring counties. However, he is too busy to serve the schools.

The local health department consists of the health officer who is over eighty years of age and has been paralyzed for several years; a public health nurse, near retirement; and a clerk. The county has not been able to recruit a sanitarian. The entire county health budget was $19,229 for fiscal 1970. Only 591 dollars was from federal sources; local appropriations covered 71 per cent of the budget.

There is no hospital in Gilmer County; the closest hospitals are up to an hour away from Glenville.* In a county where about half of the families earn less than $3,000 annually and the proportion of welfare cases is higher than the state norm, travel is too expensive for the majority. The county desperately needs transportation to out-of-county hospitals, as well as local emergency care and local practitioners.

To summarize the health problems, I would like to quote this statement by my colleague Lydia Aston, who participated in visits to rural areas:

> There are many such areas in the Appalachian region, and specifically in West Virginia, where because of lack of personal resources, inadequate public support of essential services, and unavailability of health care, significant proportions of the population have gone with-

---

*A twenty-five-bed hospital in Grantsville, Calhoun County, and a new hospital which is being built in Weston, Lewis County, to replace the present hospital facility.

out any except crisis medical care for many years. In these areas Hill-Burton built hospitals are understaffed and underused. In some of these hospitals entire wings are closed due to a shortage of physicians and nurses. County health departments in the most critical areas provide essentially no services to the county population. Well-child services and prenatal care are generally not offered in the most depressed rural areas. County public health programs in these areas are for all practical purposes phantoms on paper, with part-time health officers who are either too busy as private practitioners or too old to go to the health department routinely.[14]

ENVIRONMENTAL PROBLEMS

Except for the increased dangers of animal and insect bites and many types of rural accidents, some of these particular isolated counties have fewer environmental problems than are apparent elsewhere in West Virginia. Essentially some of the areas are undeveloped and therefore have not been defaced by strip mining. However, new permits to strip mine were issued in 1970 in five of these counties. Nineteen permits were issued in Lewis and ten in Webster Counties—signaling the initiation of gross environmental destruction in these areas. Webster is a particularly beautiful area containing 72,000 acres of state and national forest lands, and deserves to have its natural beauty protected.

Stream and air pollution is still minimal in these isolated counties. However, there is no system of solid waste disposal in most areas, resulting in a great deal of trash in the form of old cars, tin cans, stoves and refrigerators, which creates serious sight pollution.

Many of the houses in these rural areas are in poor condition leaving occupants poorly protected from heat, cold, insects, or rodents. There has been very little new construction during the last decade. Tightness of money, poor economic conditions, and apathy have resulted in minimal upkeep so that much of the housing is becoming dilapidated. In one county half of the homes lack some or all plumbing.[15] In these isolated counties only one out of four communities has a water system and only one in eight has a sewer system. Many homes lack water; sanitary facilities are crude, often leading to stream pollution.

SCHOOLS

Our conversations with physicians, dentists, and hospital administrators now living in these isolated counties brought out that one of the greatest stumbling blocks to professional recruitment is the substandard schools which exist in these areas. The school buildings are dilapidated, the curriculum is very limited and outdated, and the staff is generally poorly trained and rigid in approach. Physical punishment is permitted and even encouraged in some areas. Even in the university city of Morgantown, one day a few weeks ago a school teacher was reported to have paddled fifty-five to sixty grade school children. Some youngsters returning from home after lunch were paddled even though they did not talk in the school cafeteria, which was the alleged crime.

School bonds almost invariably fail to win community support leaving the teachers with low salaries, the buildings in disrepair, and no opportunity to revise or upgrade the curriculum. Several of the counties we visited have consolidated their high schools and are in the process of attempting to improve them. However, in one county there are still three high schools for just 635 pupils. Despite a declining population, some counties have refused to consolidate their primary schools, leaving the limited tax dollars to go for duplication instead of needed improvements.

Special programs such as those for the blind, disturbed, handicapped and retarded, and subjects such as remedial reading generally do not exist.

In addition, academic subjects are weak; vocational subjects are very limited in these rural schools, as they are throughout Appalachia, although the Appalachian Regional Commission is in the process of upgrading vocational and technical programs.[16] For example, in the eight counties there are no vocational industrial offerings in carpentry, commercial cooking, electrical work, machines, masonry, mining, and welding; in the business and office area, bookkeeping is not available at all and only three counties offer clerical and stenography courses; none of the counties offers technical vocational courses.[17] The lack of vocational training results in unskilled manpower who cannot find jobs. This is one reason why rural Appalachian people who move to urban areas find it difficult to secure a job. Furthermore, when the rural migrant does find work, he must accept the lowest-paying type of employment.

The local unskilled manpower is a stumbling block to attracting new industry to these isolated areas. In addition, the roads are too poor to accommodate commuters or to transport the goods to market. Furthermore, company officials also react negatively, the same way professionals do to poor schools, lack of health facilities, and deteriorating communities.

SOCIAL AND CULTURAL ISOLATION

Another factor mentioned as a deterrent to doctors locating in rural areas is their social and cultural isolation and the conservative and provincial attitudes of the local populace.

Poor roads, often made impassable by snow or rain, compound the social, cultural, and professional isolation faced by the health practitioners who choose to live in rural areas. On the other hand, the narrow, winding roads, often with potholes, make driving tortuously slow for the rural resident who tries to get his wife or child to a doctor or hospital. The West Virginia State Road Commission reported that in 1965 within the eight-county area only one-fifth of the road mileage met minimum specifications.[18]

Throughout West Virginia the system of public libraries is very weak. Most of these rural counties do not have libraries although a bookmobile makes infrequent rounds of some areas.

Except for Gilmer County where the State College is located, there is just nothing to do—no movie theatres except for a few drive-ins operated during the summer. Some of these counties have no motels and very few restaurants. As liquor cannot be sold by the drink except in private clubs, these areas do not have open bars. Dave Hall reports that even the former fairgrounds area, the scene of county fairs, horse and automobile racing, and other spectacles, is now closed.[19] The "major" entertainment is often a run-down poolroom or, for the men, hunting and fishing.

The local population appears to be either apathetic or hopeless about improving the situation in these areas. Even a State

Senator we spoke to could offer no hope for improving the economic picture in his county. The local banker told us there had been no new construction in years and that he had recently turned down a loan request to build a motel and restaurant from a group which included a physician. He said his bank would take no risks in the community. It should be noted that this particular town once had a large tourist trade including a 300-room hotel which had facilities for bowling, stables, tennis, and other sports.

Professor Richard Ball of West Virginia University, in a perceptive overview of the Southern Appalachian subculture, states that "resignation, apathy, and fatalism are rarely so prominent as among the members of the mountain-folk subculture."[20] Although Professor Ball is referring primarily to the poor, there appear to be some of these attitudes among other segments of the Appalachian population.

CONCLUDING COMMENTS

My task was to present the health problems of isolated Appalachian counties. The health problems are intertwined with other problems of rural and mountain areas—isolation, poverty, and the level of living. In a few counties, there were community groups attempting to attract industry or to improve the availability of health care. However, massive federal help is needed if we are to improve living conditions in rural areas.

Many people, including the President, politicians, and patriots, have expressed concern for the small group of American soldiers who are prisoners-of-war. Why can't this same concern be extended to veterans and the families of soldiers living in the ghettoes and the hills of Appalachia?

Every time I hear about a helicopter being shot down, I think of its misuse, for the helicopters destroyed in Vietnam alone could furnish all the necessary transportation for doctors into the Appalachian rural areas and transportation out for patients needing emergency care. The war demonstrates that this country has the capacity to move physicians, dentists, nurses, and indeed, entire hospitals to the rural areas of Southeast Asia. Why can't this health capacity be directed toward the rural areas of our own country?

I regret my report has been a sad one and I am tempted to brighten it with some solutions. However, I will leave that to others. Instead, I would like to close by reading from a poet who has caught my daughter's fancy, Richard Brautigan:

The Memoirs of Jesse James
I remember all those thousands of hours
that I spent in grade school watching the clock,
waiting for recess or lunch or to go home.
Waiting: for anything but school.
My teachers could easily have ridden with Jesse James
for all the time they stole from me.[21]

REFERENCES

1. Caudill, Rebecca: *My Appalachia.* New York, Holt, Rinehart and Winston, Third Printing, August 1969, p. 2.
2. Photiadis, John D.: *West Virginians in Their Own State and in Cleveland, Ohio.* Appalachian Center Information Report 3, West Virginia University, Morgantown, West Virginia, February 1970.
3. Leyden, Dennis R. and Rader, Robert D.: *County Personal Income, West Virginia, 1962-1965.* West Virginia University Economic Development Services, Number 11, Bureau of Business Research, December 1968.
4. Telephone communication between John McMillan, Department of Employment Security, Charleston, West Virginia, and Mrs. Norene Thieme, June 4, 1971.
5. Miernyk, William H.: "Economic Characteristics of Appalachia and Potential for Financing Health Care Improvements." Paper presented at Conference on Appalachian and Rural Health. *See Chapter 3.*
6. Miernyk, William H.: *Ibid.*
7. Personal communication from David Hall, April, 1971.
8. Information Center, Office of Economic Opportunity: "Community Profile Project." Computer Printout, OEO, Charleston, W. Va., December, 1970.
9. Information Center, Office of Economic Opportunity: *Ibid.*
10. Roemer, Milton I.: "Health Needs and Services of the Rural Poor." In, Report of the President's National Advisory Commission on Rural Poverty: *Rural Poverty in the United States.* USGPO, Washington, D. C., May, 1968, pp. 311-332.
11. Steinman, David: Health in rural poverty: Some lessons in theory and from experience. *Am J Public Health, 60:*1813-1823, September 1970.
12. Telephone communication between Mrs. Avis Moore, Clay County Court Clerk, and Mrs. Norene M. Thieme, June 2, 1971.
13. Sizer, Leonard M.: *County Study Data Book, Measures of Social Change*

in West Virginia, 1940-1965. West Virginia University Bulletin, Agricultural Experiment Station and Office of Research and Development, Center for Appalachian Studies and Development, West Virginia University, Morgantown, West Virginia June 1967, Table 2A, p. 64.

14. Aston, Lydia: Suggestions for Implementing the Emergency Health Personnel Act of 1970. Report to Community Health Services, HSMHA, April 1971.

15. Bureau of the Census, U. S. Department of Commerce: *1970 Census of Housing: Advance Report HC (VI)-50.* U. S. Department of Commerce, January 1971.

16. Excerpt of Hearings before Subcommittee on Economic Development of the U. S. Senate Committee on Public Works: Testimony supports continuation of Appalachian program. *Appalachia, 4:*6, March-April, 1971.

17. State Department of Education: Vocational Offerings in West Virginia Secondary Schools, 1969-1970. Charleston, West Virginia.

18. Sizer: *County Study Data Book.* Section 7, Tables 3A and 3B, pp. 82-83.

19. Hall, Op cit.,: Personal communication.

20. Ball, Richard A.: A poverty case: The analgesic subculture of the southern Appalachians. *Am Sociol Rev, 33:*892, December 1968.

21. Brautigan, Richard: The Memoirs of Jesse James. In *Rommell Drives on Deep Into Egypt.* New York, Dell Publishing Co., 1970, p. 4.

Chapter 3

ECONOMIC CHARACTERISTICS OF APPALACHIA AND POTENTIAL FOR FINANCING HEALTH CARE IMPROVEMENTS

WILLIAM H. MIERNYK

THE PUBLIC VIEW OF APPALACHIA

A LITTLE OVER A DECADE AGO the American public became aware of the existence of Appalachia. The West Virginia primary election of 1960 not only propelled John F. Kennedy into the White House, but also brought reporters from the metropolitan press into the most serious depressed region in the nation. Ten years later, other newspapermen have returned to the region and to their dismay they have discovered that poverty is still to be found in Appalachia. A half-page article by Ben A. Franklin in *The New York Times* (November 29, 1970) was headlined "Years of Vast Aid Bring Scant Relief to Appalachia." On January 27 of this year, the *Wall Street Journal* featured a front page story headlined "King Coal Booms Again But Life Remains Hard in Boone County, W. Va." A subhead states that "gloom and poverty persist despite miners' comeback. . ." The same paper recently reviewed *The Hollow* by Bill Surface (Coward-McConn, 1970) under the headline "In a Kentucky Hollow Life Goes On—Barely" (February 23, 1971). Somewhat earlier, in November, 1967, the *Washington Post* ran a long feature article under the heading "The Jelly Hasn't Helped Appalachia."

These references cover a small sample of journalistic evaluations of the current state of the Appalachian economy. I have singled them out because they were published in three of the more influential newspapers of the country. The picture they portray is one of failure. A favorite whipping boy of the reporters is the Appalachian Regional Commission which administers the Appalachian Regional Development Act. The program launched by this Act was originally scheduled to expire in June, 1971 but it has been given a four-year extension by Congress. It is surprising that this extension was granted in view of the bad press which the Appalachian Regional Development Program has received.

The regional press has done little to offset the views published by metropolitan area journalists. Appalachians are evidently self-conscious about regional poverty, and economic depression is pretty much taken for granted. Thus the public view, both within and outside the region, is one of an essentially stagnant regional economy.

What does all this have to do with the delivery of health services to rural areas in Appalachia? Actually, a great deal. Health and economic well-being are not independent. Being poor does not necessarily mean that one will be ill, and having money does not guarantee good health. In general, however, there is a direct correlation between per capita income and various health indicators. Thus economic growth, that is, rising per capita income, should lead to general improvement in basic health conditions. Finally, there has been a tendency in this country to look to federal agencies for means to provide service to rural areas. This will no doubt continue, but the problems of rural health will be dealt with more quickly, and probably more effectively, by joint federal, state and local efforts.

WHAT DID THE APPALACHIAN REGIONAL COMMISSION HOPE TO ACCOMPLISH?

The Appalachian Development Act of 1965 resulted from the recommendations made by the President's Appalachian Regional Committee (PARC) which was chaired by Franklin D. Roosevelt, Jr. This Committee drew on the Center for Regional Economic Study at the University of Pittsburgh for staff assistance in making an intensive, although necessarily abbreviated, study of the region. The Committee's report corroborated earlier impressions of dire distress in the area.

The major cause of this distress was the precipitous decline in coal production and employment between 1947 (when coal production reached a peak of 630 million tons) and 1961. During this fourteen-year interval coal production dropped by 36 per cent, and coal employment declined by 64 per cent. Two hundred seventy thousand coal miners were permanently displaced from their jobs. The major cause of the decline in coal production was a shift in demand to other types of fuel, and the drop in employment was accelerated by the famous "mechanization agreement" negotiated by John L. Lewis in 1950. The decline of agriculture employment, a nation-wide phenomenon, also had an impact on job opportunities in parts of the region. The Committee report also noted some paradoxical conditions. Appalachia, they found, was not an underindustrialized region despite its earlier dependence on extractive industries. Also, while the region was relatively well-served by railroads, essential to the movement of coal, it was not linked to the rest of the nation by an adequate system of highways. Large parts of the region had only a nominal acquaintance with the automobile age.

As a consequence of these findings, the President's Committee recommended a major highway construction program to supplement the nationwide interstate highway system. Thus, about 80 per cent of all funds authorized during the initial five years of the Appalachian Regional Development Program was for the construction of highways. An equal amount was appropriated by the thirteen states included in the region as their matching share. This meant that state funds were diverted from other uses.

Some economists have been highly critical of the emphasis on highways. They feel that the money would have been better spent directly on human resources, that is, on education and health services. They have argued that a better educated and healthier population would find it easier to obtain jobs and, if necessary, to migrate out of the region. They pointed out, quite accurately, that large parts of rural Appalachia are not economically viable, and that the best thing that could be done for the people of these subregions is to encourage them to leave.

My own view is that the critics of the Appalachian Regional Development Highways were wrong. If the region is to have an economic future, it must have an adequate transportation system, and transportation should have the highest time priority.* The region should be well along the road to an adequate system of interstate highways in three or four years as the roads now under construction are completed.

The debate of highway versus human resources investment is now of academic interest, since the highway program has gone too far to be reversed. The funds committed to it could not be diverted to other resources. It is important to recognize that in the system of development, highways represented only the first phase of the Appalachian Regional Development Program. The emphasis during the next four years will be shifted almost entirely to education and health.

WHAT HAS BEEN THE RECORD OF ACCOMPLISHMENT?

The journalistic appraisals mentioned earlier are based on the impressions of reporters who visit a few communities in the region. A more detailed statistical analysis shows a somewhat different picture. Between 1950 and 1960, net out-migration from Appalachia amounted to 2.2 million persons. During the next decade the total dropped by one-half, and the region lost only 1.1 million persons due to out-migration.

It is widely assumed that the total population of Appalachia is declining. This is not so. Between 1950 and 1960, the total population of the region increased by 2 per cent, and during the past decade by 2.7 per cent. These figures are, of course, far below the national growth rates of 18.5 and 13.3 per cent for these two decades, but the region does have a growing population.

Population growth does not necessarily mean economic growth. And it clearly does not by itself represent an increase in welfare. Per capita personal income is the most widely-used indicator of economic growth. The per capita income of Appalachia increased less than the national average during the long period of

---

*This does not mean that additional highways in the region should be given equal priority. The 632 mile Allegheny Parkway recently proposed by Senator Byrd would have little economic impact on the region and should be given a low development priority.

declining coal production and employment. It has increased at a slightly more rapid rate than that of the nation as a whole in recent years. In 1965, before the Appalachian Regional Development Program was in operation, Appalachia's per capita income of 2,147 dollars amounted to 77.7 per cent of national per capita income. Three years later, in 1968, the gap had been narrowed slightly, and per capita income in Appalachia stood at 78.8 per cent of the national average. This may appear to be a small gain, but considering the brevity of the period involved it must be recognized as a significant gain. Furthermore, when the data for 1969 and 1970 are compiled on a regional basis there should be a further narrowing of this gap.

In two of the four years for which data are available since the Appalachian Regional Commission was established, employment in the region has gone up faster than in the nation as a whole, but in the other two years there was a lag in the region. On balance, it is probably safe to conclude that Appalachia is maintaining its existing state in terms of employment.

Largely because of the precipitous drop of employment in coal mining, the unemployment rate in Appalachia has been above the national average since 1947. For almost two decades the gap was substantial, but there has been some narrowing of these differences since 1965. In that year the unemployment rate in Appalachia was 5.1 per cent compared to the national average of 4.5 per cent. In 1969, these rates were 3.9 per cent for Appalachia and 3.5 per cent for the United States. The 1970 data, when compiled on a regional basis, may show that the difference has been virtually eliminated.

These short-term trends indicate that there has been improvement of economic conditions in Appalachia vis-a-vis the nation since 1965. This is clear evidence of a reversal. Does it mean that the problem has been solved? If so, should the credit go entirely to the Appalachian Regional Development Program?

Clearly, the economic problems of Appalachia have not been solved. Income in the region is still well below the national average, and the official unemployment rate is somewhat above the national average. In economic terms the region is no longer slipping relative to the nation. It is gaining although only slowly. Finally, the relative improvement in regional economic conditions is due more to the revival of coal mining in the region than to organized development activities. The revival of coal is a direct consequence of the exponentially rising demand for electrical energy.

The Appalachian Regional Development Program is a long-range program. It would have been one of the major accomplishments of all time if this relatively small-scale effort had been able to accomplish all of the improvement we have observed during the past four or five years. This does not mean that the Appalachian Regional Development Program has been a failure. I would argue that it has been a success. It will be another five to ten years, however, before the effects of the highway development systems are felt in the region. It may be even longer before the region's health and educational deficiencies are overcome.

RURAL-URBAN IMBALANCE

The most striking difference between Appalachia and the rest of the United States is not to be found by comparing income, employment, or other conventional indicators of economic well-being. The major difference is in the rural-urban distribution of population. The 1970 census of population shows that 73.5 per cent of all residents in the nation live in urban places. A comparable figure is not available for Appalachia as a whole, but for West Virginia the figure is 39 per cent. More than half of the population of North and South Carolina also live in rural areas. When population data are compiled on a regional basis, they will show that most of the subregions of Appalachia are heavily rural, and that most of them are non-farm rural areas.

Why should this be considered a problem, particularly in an age when we hear so much about the "urban crisis"? The answer is that the economic advantages of rural life have been greatly exaggerated. Actually, the urban crisis has been caused by the migration of relatively uneducated, unskilled members of the population from rural areas to the cities. This is a consequence of major technological changes in agriculture and mining which have permitted us to increase output from the extractive sectors with steadily diminishing labor requirements. The poor have been transferred from rural areas, where they are largely invisible, to urban areas where they are highly visible. But, it is not my assignment to discuss the problems of cities, so I will return to the rural residents of Appalachia.

The strategy of economic development that has evolved in the Appalachian Regional Commission Program is called a "growth point" strategy. Essentially, this means the concentration of public investment in relatively large communities and particularly in communities which have growth potential. One hope is that the highway system will make it easier for these communities to grow by providing a steadily increasing number of job opportunities. The next step will be to encourage rural residents to move to the growth centers where they and their children will have access to better educational and economic opportunities. It is important to stress that the strategy is to make these rural-urban population shifts within the region. This is quite a different approach than one which would encourage Appalachian rural residents to migrate to the metropolitan areas along the East Coast or in the Midwest.

The growth point strategy is based upon two economic concepts: one of these we call "economies of scale"; the other refers to "external effects."

The notion of economies of scale is a simple one. It simply means that certain things have to be fairly large in order to be efficient. Steel, for example, cannot be produced in small shops operated by two or three men. Nor would we expect to find highly specialized medical services in a small rural clinic. Hospitals, like steel mills, are organized on the basis of economies of scale even if we do not use dollars as the measure of efficiency.

The notion of externalities is a little more complicated, particularly since there are both positive and negative externalities. In nontechnical terms, a positive externality is something that happens outside a given organization which has a favorable influence on the internal operation of that organization. The notion of externalities may be applied to communities as well as to an industrial firm.

The location of a factory in a community will provide jobs and presumably will lead to higher income. It may do more than that. It could create a demand for additional health facilities. A new hospital might be built in the community. Additional skills might also be brought to the community as a result of the factory. All of these effects could attract other kinds of economic activity. If enough factories are built in the community, suppliers of various kinds of intermediate goods and business services will locate there. This will stimulate other kinds of growth external to the production process. This, in a nutshell, is how cities get started and how cities grow.

The advantages of a growth point strategy may be evident to the residents of communities where public investments are made, but how can they possibly help the rural areas? The growth point strategy does not mean that the needs of rural residents will be ignored. But, these needs should be satisfied in a way which will not discourage the long-run shift from rural to urban areas that must take place if Appalachia is to move closer to national averages in terms of employment, unemployment, wages, and income.

WHERE WILL THE ECONOMIC DEVELOPMENT OF APPALACHIA OCCUR?

It is evident from the above comments that the economic development of Appalachia is not expected to be spatially uniform. Most of this development will take place in a limited number of urban places and in their surrounding hinterland areas. To put the matter bluntly, large sections of rural Appalachia will not benefit directly or indirectly from the projected economic growth of the region. This is not, incidentally, a uniquely Appalachian phenomenon. Most of the rural counties of America are not growing, but in other parts of the country the rural-to-urban population adjustment appears to go on more smoothly (and more rapidly) than it does in Appalachia.

I will not attempt in this short chapter to identify all of the "growth centers" of Appalachia, but I will illustrate my point by referring to the outlook for West Virginia. There are four growth areas in this state that are fairly easy to identify. These are the following: the Eastern Panhandle; an area extending along Interstate 79 from Morgantown on the north to Weston on the south; the Ohio Valley, particularly between Huntington and Parkersburg; and at a somewhat later date, the area between Huntington and Charleston. These are the places where industrial and commercial expansion will take place, where new job opportunities will be created, and where there are places that will absorb the out-migrants who leave rural counties but remain in West Virginia. The remaining counties, and this means a substantial majority, are not expected to grow. The Charleston area and the Northern Panhandle are fairly congested, and the lack of suitable land for further economic development is already a constraint. But, the other parts of West Virginia are not expected to grow because they do not have viable economic bases. As in West Virginia, the economic outlook for most of these remaining parts of rural Appalachia remains bleak.

COMPREHENSIVE HEALTH SERVICE NETWORKS

The health service networks, which the Appalachian Regional Commission has proposed and started to implement, are designed to improve the quality of health services available to rural Appalachians without major investment in immoble facilities in areas outside the growth centers. The notion is a simple one. It is to construct a hierarchy of medical facilities built around a central Regional Hospital Complex. The Regional Complex will be linked to local general hospitals and these in turn are tied to local community health centers by a health referral and emergency transport network. The comprehensive health network is, of course, a long-term goal. Meanwhile, the Commission has sponsored a number of Health Demonstration Programs. One of the unique features of these programs is that they were designed to demonstrate "the value of adequate health facilities and services for the *economic development* of the region" (Appalachia, January, 1971, p. 11, emphasis added). It may be difficult to do this because of the problems of measurement, but no one has yet questioned the assumption that improved health services will contribute to the economic development of the residents of the region.

As the regional development program has progressed, there has been a growing emphasis on preventive health care. It is believed by some members of the Commission's Health Advisory Committee that the best preventive health care is the elimination of poverty. Those who have advanced this view believe that with a rise in per capita income many of the health deficiencies attributable to malnutrition will be eliminated.

The Commission is now planning an expansion of prenatal and maternal care programs, as well as programs to ensure adequate nourishment for children from birth to maturity. By eliminating health deficiencies traceable to malnutrition, the Commission hopes to improve the educational performance of rural Appalachians. A healthier and better educated population, they reason, will provide a long-run solution to the problems of poverty in this region. To date, I have heard no one question either the goal or the method of reaching this objective.

Doctors, especially those concerned with public health, are inclined to relate the need for medical facilities to the need for medical care in specific areas. The poor are generally more in need of medical care than those who are able to support adequate diets and medical treatment when required. The difficult question is how to provide medical care in declining rural areas without major investment in fixed medical facilities. From an economic point of view there is only one answer, which may not be a tenable answer, considering the life-style preferences of doctors and other medical personnel.

Rural areas should be served by mobile health facilities and personnel. Investment in hospitals, clinics, and other medical facilities should be restricted to urban centers with reasonable economic growth prospects. This is the only way to take advantage of economies of scale and positive externalities while at the same time providing at least minimal health care for those who do not live within easy traveling distance of a hospital.

This conclusion may not satisfy anyone's humanitarian instincts. But, it is one that is easy to support by conventional benefit-cost analysis. If the health needs of the rural poor in Appalachia are to be met during a transitional period, a large number of mobile medical personnel will be required. What rural Appalachia needs is a corps of domestic "medical missionaries" willing to forego, at least temporarily, the conveniences and comforts of urban life. Mobile health facilities should be able to provide minimal health care to rural Appalachians without slowing down the long-run transition from a predominantly rural to a predominantly urban society.

CONCLUSIONS

At the end of the five years, one is able to observe that genuine progress has been made in stimulating economic development in Appalachia. None of the goals of the Appalachian Regional Commission has been reached as yet, but no one could have realistically expected them to be reached by now. The entire health program is still in its infancy, but the provision of health services should be considerably accelerated within the next four years. None of this means that the problems of Appalachia are almost solved.

The economic progress that has been made in Appalachia has been largely limited to the region's urban counties. There have been few spillover benefits to rural, non-farm counties. These recent trends are expected to continue, and a comprehensive program of health care should take them into account.

Finally, evaluation of the economic development of Appalachia must be conducted within a reasonable time frame. The newspapermen who come to Appalachia and discover that poverty has not been eliminated remind one of the California native who wrote to his Congressman six months after the latter had taken office for the first time. In his list of complaints the constituent included the following: "When you were running for election you promised that the Sierras would be reforested. You have been in office for six months now, and the mountains still are not covered with trees."

Chapter 4

HEALTH CARE BARRIERS IN APPALACHIA

G. David Steinman

Individuals need and value several elements when they seek medical help for themselves or their dependents: first, someone knowledgeable in matters of disease, treatment, and prognosis; second, one who can take action; and third, a medical trustee—one to be engaged to care for the individual and hence to understand him in the context of his life. As we know, significant casual factors of pathology exist in the environment around us. A competent health professional would initiate preventive steps before the symptom stage that brings the patient to seek attention. This implies a continuing relationship.

Bloom has described the doctor-patient relationship as one where expressive and instrumental transaction is carried out between the two parties. The patient is surrounded behaviorally by his family, and in turn by their subcultural reference groups, and finally, the dominant sociocultural matrix. This matrix contains the doctor enclosed in his profession, and his subcultural reference groups.[1]

Appalachian subculture greets the traditionally trained professional with characteristics widely discussed and some as yet unnoted. Jack Weller, author of *Yesterday's People*, has portrayed Appalachian life style in a somewhat atypical four-act drama:

Act One describes the terrain—the impossibly vast barrier of ridge after ridge separating narrow valleys which form "hollows" in their cul-de-sacs. Road distance often more than doubles distance by air.

Act Two focuses on the settlers of this region. Many were runaway Anglo-Saxon workers from Virginia plantations. Here they remained, in the side waters of the road to the West through the

Cumberland Gap. The region was border country in the Civil War and became important only as coal and lumber were searched out largely in the early twentieth century.

Act Three sees the mountaineer's socioeconomic fate sealed as he sold out his lumber and coal holdings to outside sources.

In Act Four present attributes of the population are enumerated as consequences of this lack of opportunity.

Middle Class	*Mountaineer*
1. Middle class America equates effort with success.	1. The mountaineer has failed in spite of his efforts.
2. Our dads started at the bottom and worked up.	2. Mr. Combs or Caudle or Maynard started at the bottom and stayed at the bottom.
3. We know education pays and we pay for education.	3. The mountaineer is yet to be convinced of the value of education.
4. We measure the achievement factor. We search for role fulfillment.	4. Middle class American role fulfillment is not possible. Family interaction is where the mountaineer seems to find meaning.

More insight into this state can be gained by a portion of Charles Reich's *Greening of America.*

Appalachia is associated with an extractive and agricultural economy, with poorly developed systems of schools and roads. Isolation, more than any other single condition, characterizes the rural poor and distinguishes them from the more fortunate segments of rural America. The most extreme conditions of rural poverty involve three kinds of isolation: geographic, economic, and cultural.[2]

A higher incidence of several disease states can be expected in populations of rural poor. In addition, available medical resources are generally lacking in both quantity and quality.

The increased assault on health stems from factors in the general environment and from the nature of occupational hazards. The environment is characterized by contaminated water and inadequate sewage disposal. Inadequate housing and clothing result in increased exposure. Furthermore, mining and farming are two of the most dangerous occupations in the United States. Only the construction industry suffers a higher death rate. Decreased resistance is, in part, accounted for by the crowding of large families in small homes, by poor nutrition, and by lack of proper clothing. These factors are perpetuated by a tendency to marry young and have large families.

Although rural families in America have been shown to have greater general medical needs than do urban families, they are often disadvantaged in the care they receive. Distance from facilities, costs, and attitudes are involved. Rural physicians and nurses are generally older, less specialized, and less informed about current practices. There are relatively fewer professional health workers in rural populations.

People in the southern Appalachian region have traditionally been stereotyped as being strongly fatalistic. When present, this trait would tend to diminish the perceived seriousness of a given condition in terms of stimulus to take action. With regard to the place of health in the value hierarchy of an individual, Koos found that both family traditions and social class influenced the place of health. Health as a value often finds itself displaced downward by other strivings.[3] Several studies have shown health needs to be superseded by jobs, housing, education, and police protection.[4]

TABLE 4-I

FACTORS DETERMINING HEALTH AND ILLNESS BEHAVIOR

Perceived Threat	*Perceived Value of Action*
Perceived susceptibility	Perceived probability that action produces results
Perceived seriousness	Cost of action
Importance of health	Past utilization of medical services

Appalachian attitudes toward scientific medicine were illustrated as follows: when asked if a physician could "look you over without doing tests and find everything important," eight per cent of the people said "yes," 85 per cent said "no" and 7 per cent "did not know." However, although 73 per cent of the heads of households felt that a good health checkup would be worth more than 15 dollars, only 25 per cent said they would pay that and more than 50 per cent said they would pay nothing at all. Therefore, while periodic health checkups performed in a scientific way are seen to be of value, the typical household cannot afford this. Private funds would be spent for such services in a minority of the households of this population.

The nature of health practices also influences quality of care. The response to illness has been said to lead a person to one of four alternative systems, i.e. a) modern medicine, b) faith medicine, c) folk medicine, or d) pseudo medicine.[5] In several studies, both urban and rural poor have been shown to utilize decreased amounts of scientific services. Folk medicine and faith medicine frequently conflict with medical science when dependence upon them involves delaying or neglecting to take advantage of scientific responses to serious disease.

In Martin County the households did not seem to differ much from the middle class. More than 50 per cent of households there had analgesics, liniments, laxatives, and insecticides. Fewer than 25 per cent of these households had "kidney pills, blood tonic, or liver pills." The use of home remedies made from leaves, bark, and roots was explored. Only 5 per cent of the families had such home remedies for colds and stomach complaints. Other remedies were used by fewer than a dozen households in the total sample of 2,190 households.

Further insight into the health and illness behavior of the mountain poor was obtained by an analysis of nonrespondents to several programs. In Leslie County, 751 households were selected for multiphasic screening. There were 489 respondents and 262 nonrespondents. Of the respondents, 208 families responded in total and 281 gave partial response. Of the 281, the husband was the absent member in 151 incidents, the wife in 70, and other family members in 60.

Of the nonrespondents, a sample was selected and interviews were carried out to determine factors associated with nonresponse. Twenty-five per cent had been unable to attend because of present family illness. Twenty per cent had conflicting job responsibilities. Fourteen per cent preferred their own physician. Seven per cent claimed they had received no communication about the clinic. Eleven per cent had inadequate transportation. Six per cent believed that the family was healthy and did not need a health checkup. Five per cent were afraid that the exam would reveal illnesses. Five per cent had lost or forgotten the date of scheduling. Two per cent disapproved of the project. Two per cent did not attend because of inclement weather, and two per cent feared the examination would be physically painful. In summary, major organizational reasons were: family illness, 35 per cent; job responsibilities, 28 per cent; no letter received, 10 per cent; and no transportation, 17 per cent. Attitudinal reasons included preference of own physician in 49 per cent of the cases, belief that the family was healthy and not in need of a checkup in 21 per cent, fear that the examination would reveal illness in 16 per cent, disapproval of the project in 7 per cent, and fear of physical examination in 7 per cent of the cases.[6]

The provider faces formidable hazards in delivering health care in Appalachia. An appreciation for these factors can be found in a study done in the Department of Behavioral Science at the University of Kentucky several years ago.[7] The study population included some one hundred physicians who had left practice in Eastern Kentucky. The most frequent reasons given were the following: dissatisfaction of physician's wife with isolation and small town life; dissatisfaction with public schools; and the feeling that excessive demands on practice with inadequate resources resulted in deteriorating standards of care.

Since that time Regina McCormick, working in Virginia, has interviewed physicians leaving primary care practice. More than seventy were interviewed.[8] Measures which respondents felt would be of benefit in enhancing a primary care practice included the following: group practice, 96 per cent; residency programs in primary practice, 81 per cent; association with residents and medical students, 74 per cent; tax incentives for physicians devoted to primary care, 69 per cent; nurse practitioners or physician assistants, 66 per cent; prepayment or guaranteed income, 49 per cent; and direct subsidy to the practice from the community, 46 per cent.

New emphasis must be given to continuing and comprehensive care; the family must be understood and approached as a basic service unit. However, the growing complexity of medical resources, while increasing medicine's efficiency in healing, requires the integrated function of the extended health team. There often is not enough time for the physician to individually gather the data and/or give the needed "human" response to the patient. He cannot remember all that his patients have told him, or what his clinical findings and treatments were. He does not have the time for inquiring further into some obvious areas of concern. The above indicates two basic needs: the provision of adequate information for clinical analysis, payment, and medicolegal problems and assistance in working-up and caring for patients.[9]

We, at a University of Kentucky demonstration clinic, the Clover Fork Clinic at Evarts, Kentucky, put these leads together and came up with a model: a satellite clinic, staffed with two physicians during the day and nurse practitioners, radio, and ambulance facilities around the clock, backed up by a regional hospital, with its emergency room, a full complement of specialists, and other outreach programs. We are presently in our tenth month of operation.

What about the larger view? American medicine has been criticized as an unplanned venture, implying lack of coordination and shared priorities. These barriers to the delivery of health care in Appalachia are being attacked by the Appalachian Regional Commission. The program for the Kentucky Demonstration Area is stated as follows:

> . . .The goal has been translated into a set of tangible program objectives. The five objectives comprising this set provide the basis for the definition and presentation of the project and set forth what the project is designed to demonstrate. These objectives are as follows:
>
> 1. Development and operation of a coordinated system for emergency care.
> 2. Development and operation of a coordinated system of supportive services for the chronically ill and disabled not in institutions.
> 3. Development and operation of a coordinated system of levels of care (acute, extended, long-term, and ambulatory) with balance among facilities for the various levels and functional relationships for continuity of care to achieve appropriate utilization in all sections of the region.

4. Development and operation of a coordinated system of community services for promotion and improvement of health.
5. Development and operation of a coordinated system for improving environmental conditions which jeopardize health.

These objectives are further defined in terms of program elements which must be developed to reach each objective. Requirements for facilities, equipment, and financing of services have been derived for each of the respective objectives by projecting the program elements requisite to it with provision for the phasing of their development.[10]

The need for and benefit of such large sector planning activity has been demonstrated. We are aware that health problems of the poor were intertwined with social and welfare problems to the extent that provision of adequate services for one condition or one area, in the face of several known defects, actually serves to reinforce feelings of frustration. In our Martin County experience a real need existed for more broadly based referral sources, but these did not exist. Due to the extremely fragmented nature of referral services, representatives of the state and local agencies of Kentucky, of the University of Kentucky Medical Center, and personnel of the local comprehensive health project were brought together at the invitation of the Governor's Office. The purpose was to centralize referral procedures; obtain full-time referral personnel with training; and experiment with a new working relationship between health and welfare programs. It was decided that the scope of services would be confined to the health area.

In this remote county with no full-time physicians, 1,600 people, or about 50 per cent of the 3,354 screened, were seen in the referral center. Twenty-four per cent of the infants seen were referred, as were 49 per cent of the childrn and 61 per cent of the adults. Seventy-four per cent of the referrals were made for diagnostic services and 10 per cent for direct care by a physician. Many multiple referrals were made. The average number of conditions per person was 2.2. Twenty-eight per cent had one problem, 37 per cent had two problems, 22 per cent had three problems, and 13 per cent had four or more problems.

It was found that 66 per cent of the referees relied on income resources other than their own earned wages. Of the individuals seen, only 11 per cent were in households making more than 300 dollars per month. In this situation, it was found that public institutions were utilized in 89 per cent of all referrals. Six hundred fifty-five complete referrals were made to special diagnostic clinics financed by the health project, 118 to public institutions, and 109 to other public programs. Thus, the private sector was used in only 11 per cent of all complete referrals: 116 to private physicians, 54 to private doctors of dental science, and 5 to voluntary health agencies. The most common conditions requiring referral were dental (22%) ; eye (12%) ; ear, nose and throat (9%) ; gastrointestinal (6%) ; genitourinary (5%) ; cardiac (5%) ; and behavioral (4%).

Only 47 percent of all referrals made were completed, compared to 49 per cent of the referrals made for the six-year-old children in the thirteen counties. The easiest referrals to complete were for psychiatry, dentistry, family planning, and handicapped children.

A survey was again made of those individuals who did not complete referrals. Motivational factors accounted for 67.6 per cent of the uncompleted referrals, and organization of medical care accounted for only 32 per cent. Among the 829 considered to have been deterred by motivational factors, 77 were thought to be unable to understand the reason for medical referral. Two hundred and thirty-eight simply did not value the need for care and said they would "take care of the problem later." The remainder had other motivational problems. Among the 393 with organization problems, lack of transportation was a cause in 130 cases and lack of funds to finance care in 116. The resource agencies did not follow through in 43 cases, and other organization problems were responsible in 108 instances.[11]

In summary, formidable barriers exist in both the receipt of and the delivery of medical care to all sections of Appalachia. A strong case can be made for the place of the community process as an important approach in overcoming these problems. This process is implied in the following statement:

> Successful programs to attain health goals involve effective organization and delivery of health services and the responsible utilization of these services by their [users]. Each of these, in turn, requires de-

cisions and actions by people—by the providers and [users] of health services, and by those who control the availability of resources—legal, economical, and political.[12]

There is ample opportunity and challenge in a multiplicity of roles and efforts for better health care in Appalachia. Overcoming barriers is an action role. We must will to proceed.

REFERENCES

1. Bloom, Samuel W.: *The Doctor and His Patient.* New York, The Free Press, 1965, p. 256.
2. Straus, R.: Poverty as an obstacle to health progress in our rural areas. *Am J Public Health, 55, 11:*1772, November, 1965.
3. Koos, E.: *The Health of Regionville.* Columbia University Press, 1963.
4. Notkin, H. and Notkin, M.: Community participation in health services: A review article. *Med Care Rev, 27, 11:*1178, December, 1970.
5. Straus, R.: Sociological determinants of health beliefs and behavior. *Am J Public Health, 51, 10:*1547, October, 1961.
6. Steinman, D.: Health in rural poverty: Some lessons in theory and from experience. *Am J Public Health, 60, 9:*1814, September 1970.
7. Enroth, Ronald M.: *Patterns of Response to Rural Medical Practice and Rural Life in Eastern Kentucky.* Unpublished Ph.D. thesis, University of Kentucky, 1967.
8. Crawford, R. L. and McCormack, R. C.: Reasons physicians leave primary practice. *J Med Ed, 46, 4:*263, April, 1971.
9. Clover Fork Clinic, Evarts, Kentucky: Unpublished statement of Medical Care Focus.
10. *Southeastern Kentucky Regional Health Demonstration Project.* August, 1967 edition, Lexington, Kentucky.
11. *Health Status of the Population of Martin County, Kentucky, 1964-1965.* Unpublished, Department of Community Medicine, University of Kentucky.
12. Author unknown.

Chapter 5

HEALTH CARE FOR RURAL PEOPLE: SOLUTIONS ATTEMPTED AROUND THE WORLD

Milton I. Roemer

RURAL HEALTH PROBLEMS

Deficiencies in health services among rural populations are found in every country of the world. In the poorest countries to the richest, in the most agricultural and underdeveloped to the most industrialized and highly developed, the rural population tends to receive a lower level of health service in relation to its needs than the urban. This is found both by quantitative measures of services utilized and by estimates of the quality of those services.

Striking evidence for this has recently been produced by a national study in Columbia, South America, where a higher incidence of sickness was found among rural people in household surveys (both interviews and medical examinations) than among urban; yet, there was a lower volume of ambulatory and hospital services received by rural people, even counting the ministrations of nonscientific healers. In the developing countries generally, the village-dweller gets a higher proportion of his limited volume of medical care from traditional healers than does the city-dweller; he also depends more heavily on self-prescribed drugs. In the United States, the mortality rates among rural people are somewhat lower among urban, but the volume of sickness, especially chronic, is higher; the utilization of ambulatory medical and dental services and of hospitalization is distinctly lower.

To cope with these inequities, almost all countries have undertaken special efforts to compensate for the inherent handicaps of the rural environment. These efforts are nearly always put forth at the national level. It seems to be generally recognized that the solution of rural health care problems must be like the treatment of a systemic disease; the rural symptom is only a manifestation of a systemic disorder, and to alleviate or cure it, actions must be taken to modify the functioning of the total system.

For the sake of brevity, I should like to oversimplify a very diversified array of social actions to cope with rural health care problems, and consider them under eight categories. In practice, actions in each of these spheres are obviously interrelated to actions in the other spheres, and the overall effort is heavily influenced by the general sociopolitical design of the health service system. Yet, it is interesting to observe how much consistency exists in certain types of health measurement even among countries at different points on the political spectrum and at different stages of economic development.

PREVENTION OF DISEASE

The prevention of disease or promotion of health through environmental or mass population measures figures prominently in rural health improvement efforts everywhere. In the developing countries, vector-borne diseases, like malaria or schistosomiasis, are highly prevalent in rural populations and are the object of environmental control campaigns. These are usually launched by central governments, filling in swamps, spraying houses with insecticides, eliminating snails from streams, etc., even when there is a local health agency available for personal health services. Improvements in rural water supplies and excreta disposal systems have been a very slow process and, in the developing countries, have usually depended on provision of equipment and technical aid from central Ministries of Health.

The most widespread preventive efforts in personal health service have been in the promotion of maternal and child health. The periodic examination of the expectant woman and the checkup of the small baby, with immunizations, advice on proper feeding, and hygienic counselling are a staple of rural health programs in Latin America, Asia, and Africa, as much as in Europe and North America. In the developing world, both the examinations and advice are typically provided by midwives and other auxiliary personnel, rarely by doctors. Moreover, in these countries, the sharp distinction between prevention and treatment applied in the United States is seldom found in rural programs (though it persists in the larger cities) ; the sick baby is treated to the extent possible. A common program in rural health centers is the rehydration (through parenteral fluids) of infants dehydrated from gastrointestinal disease. The effectiveness of these MCH programs is reflected by the decline almost everywhere of rural infant mortality rates over the last thirty or forty years, even though they generally remain higher than the urban.

Reduced infant mortality has led in many countries of Asia and Africa, less so in Latin America, to another form of prevention, family planning. With declines in death rates, population growth has accelerated. The large field of population control and family planning cannot be discussed here, except to note that in India, Thailand, Ghana, and elsewhere, contraceptive programs have been incorporated within the rural MCH activities. Insertions of intra-uterine devices and male sterilization procedures are performed by doctors, but dispensing of pills and contraceptive instructions of other types are usually carried out by rural nurses or midwives. Chile, under its new Marxist government, seems to be the first Latin American country to incorporate family planning into its national health policy.

GETTING DOCTORS TO RURAL AREAS

Concentrations of doctors in the large cities are worldwide phenomena. To some extent, of course, this is quite reasonable, insofar as cities must be centers for serving large regions with highly specialized care. The resultant shortages of doctors in the small towns serving rural districts are often severe and a variety of corrective actions have been taken.

Most basic has been the expansion everywhere of medical schools, so as to produce a greater national output of doctors. As long as the national supply is deficient, the rural areas with their general cultural handicaps will attract the fewest medical graduates. The most impressive increases in the total output of doctors have occurred in the Soviet Union and other socialist countries. Cuba, for example, has much more than made up for its massive exodus of doctors following the 1959 revolution; it now has over 7,000 doctors for its 8,000,000 people—a ratio (about 1:1150) equal to that of the Scandinavian countries a few years ago. Nearly all the Latin American countries have achieved improved ratios of doctors over the last thirty years, and the establishment of medical schools in the newly emancipated countries of Africa is doing the same.

After production of doctors, of course, the task is to bring about their distribution in relation to population needs, and various methods have been used. Since about 1935, Mexico has made a period of "social service" in a rural village a condition for earning the medical degree; originally this was for six months and now it is for a year. An increasing number of countries in Latin America and Asia are doing likewise. Indonesia and Turkey have such requirements; Iran achieves this end through a period of service in the Rural Health Corps, as a form of military obligation. Malaysia has recently instituted a two-year rural service requirement, in connection with the output of the first graduating class from its own medical school (formerly its doctors had to be trained abroad). The Soviet Union requires three years of service by new medical graduates in a rural health center.

Several states in our country have had "rural medical fellowship" programs since the 1940's, including Virginia and North Carolina. The new graduate serves a year in a rural area of need for each medical school year in which he has received fellowship support. The recently passed Emergency Health Personnel Act of 1970 is the first federal approach to the problem, using military obligation as the device for getting doctors to rural areas; appropriations for implementation of this law are still being awaited.

The tougher task is to hold doctors in rural areas after an initial period. The experience of the mandatory rural service programs, both in the United States and elsewhere, is that when the statutory obligation is fulfilled, the young doctor usually leaves for a city. In the Soviet Union, this tendency is countered by payment of higher salaries for a rural than for a comparable urban position. Similar salary differentials for rural work have recently been introduced in Mexico.

Assuring a satisfactory income is, of course, basic to the solution of the rural doctor problem. Even though earnings are obviously not the whole story, we know that in the United States, country doctor incomes are lower than those in all city-sizes except the multi-million population metropolises. Various schemes have been used to guarantee rural incomes. In the rural municipalities of the Canadian prairie provinces, salaries have been paid to general practitioners by local government since 1917. The Highlands and Islands Scheme of northern Scotland pays salaries to doctors who could not hope to make an adequate income from the sparse population in this region. New Zealand has similar arrangements in isolated localities, administered by the national Ministry of Health. Coal mining communities in West Virginia and other Appalachian states have long supported doctors through salaries paid from local employer-employee prepayment plans. The basic issue of adequate income support for doctors and others in rural health service is, of course, tied up with the general problem of economic support which will be explored below.

Other inducements besides income designed to keep doctors in rural places include provision of housing. Many American towns offer an attractive house at very low rental as an inducement. In the developing countries, government-financed housing is a standard feature or rural assignments for the doctor, along with other health personnel. Office quarters at low rentals have also been offered to doctors by small towns in Canada and the United States; many of these are small health centers built with the assistance of the Sears Roebuck Foundation. The provision of modern rural hospitals, of course, is also an attraction for doctors—a basic premise is back of the Hill-Burton hospital construction program in this country.

In Great Britain, rural settlement of doctors is encouraged by a national policy of designating certain areas as "over-doctored"; in these areas, typically metropolitan, new doctors are not permitted to settle—at least not under the financial support of the National Health Service. As a result, the doctors going elsewhere will sometimes be channeled to rural communities. There was a somewhat similar policy in West Germany, where the local sickness funds with heavy medical participation used to prohibit new doctors from entering, thereby compelling them to settle in areas of greater need; unfortunately for rural areas, a recent German court decision invalidated this policy in the interest of "free trade" for the medical profession. Tunisia, on the other hand, is a country which has banned new doctors from settling in the busy national capital, Tunis, thereby diverting them to other towns. All such policies as these obviously require national health planning and the exercise of considerable control over the flow of funds to pay for medical care.

ANCILLARY HEALTH MANPOWER

The use of personnel other than doctors to meet health needs has been more extensively applied in rural areas than in cities throughout the world. The well-known "feldsher" of Czarist Russia was originally a rural medical replacement for the doctor. After the revolution, with the great increase in doctor output, there was an intention to eliminate this type of health worker as substandard, but ultimately the feldsher was kept. He, or she, now works in both rural and urban areas as a general medical auxiliary, with wider responsibilities than the nurse; in rural posts the *feldsher* serves villages of a few hundred people—too few to warrant a full-time physician. An important feature of the Soviet manpower model is the freedom of *feldshers* or nurses to undertake further studies and become doctors—this is one of the reasons that so many Soviet doctors are women.

Many countries have trained special classes of middle-level health personnel for rural service. Ethiopia has its famous Public Health Training College at Gondar, where "health officers" are trained for both curative and preventive work in rural health centers; their curriculum requires three years of study after high school, followed by a year of supervised field work. Community nurses and sanitarians are similarly trained in relatively short periods. Venezuela has its rural program of so-called "simplified medicine," staffed by auxiliary nurses and male medical assistants.

In Ceylon, rural posts are staffed by dispensers of common remedies, who are still quaintly called "apothecaries." In Malaysia, the old British term of "hospital assistant" is applied to male health personnel who give the curative service in rural health centers, while nurses and nursing assistants give the preventive service. Throughout Africa the "dresser," a male auxiliary with very little formal schooling, is the most common source of medical care, except for primitive healers, for most of the rural population.

Most of the world's babies are undoubtedly delivered by midwives who have learned their skills simply from observation and experience. Throughout Asia and Africa, less so in Latin America, young village women with grade school education have been given formal training of one or two years to serve as "government midwives." The task everywhere is to win over the rural people to use these trained midwives, rather than the untrained ones with whom they are usually more familiar. The trained midwife, of course, is by no means limited to rural areas of underdeveloped countries. She is the attendant at most childbirths in Great Britain and Holland where the infant and maternal mortality records are, incidentally, better than in the United States.

The hundreds of millions of people in rural China have long depended on herbalists and acupuncturists for their medical care. Under the current Communist government, thousands of young peasants have been trained to offer immunizations, first-aid for injuries, scientific drugs for common diseases and education about personal hygiene. These "barefoot doctors," as they are called, are now the mainstays of rural health care in the People's Republic, working as part of a network of both Western and traditional medicine in each province.

RURAL HOSPITALS AND HEALTH CENTERS

Insofar as local wealth has financed hospital construction, rural populations have always been left behind. This has been true in the wealthy United States no less than in India or Brazil. It took the Hill-Burton Act in our country, with its strong priorities for rural states and the rural regions within every state, to improve the relative hospital bed supply for rural people. Over the last twenty-five years since this program was started, bed supply has been quite well equalized between rural and urban areas; in fact, the dynamics of patient flow today are such that the greater pressures of bed shortage are being felt in the city hospitals which are serving both urban and rural people.

Hospital construction in the main provincial towns serving rural districts is a standard objective in the Ministry of Health plans in countries of Latin America, Asia, and Africa. While urban hospitals are often built by voluntary bodies or purely private groups, rural district hospitals nearly always depend on central government; the chief exception are the hospitals, usually small, established by foreign religious missions. Throughout Latin America, and also in Iran and Turkey, social security agencies separate from Health Ministries have built many large well-equipped hospitals; these are limited, however, to their beneficiaries who are nearly always industrial or commercial workers in the main cities.

The rural district hospital outside of Western Europe and North America typically has much responsibiilty for ambulatory care. Its out-patient department provides the specialty care for the whole district, since private specialists are nonexistent in these areas. In Great Britain, all hospitals come under the control of Regional Hospital Boards which attempt to coordinate the response to needs in both cities and the rural sections around them. Sweden also has a regionalization scheme, under which graded responsibilities are assigned to rural, district, and provincial hospitals. The hospital in Chile is administratively responsible for all official health services, ambulatory and environmental, in its catchment area. This is the pattern also in the Soviet Union.

Probably more important on a world scale than the rural hospital is the rural health center—a facility for ambulatory service, curative and preventive. These are different intensities of staffing. In Mexico, for example, there are the Type A health centers, staffed by several doctors with specialty qualifications and located in the main provincial towns; the Type B centers are staffed by one general medical practitioner aided by nurses and other auxiliaries; the Type C centers in small villages are staffed only by auxiliary personnel, visited occasionally by a supervising doctor. Malaysia and Thailand have their "main health centers," staffed by one doctor and several nurses and auxiliaries, and "sub-centers," staffed only by auxiliaries. In Sub-Sahara Africa, the health centers are usually staffed only by dressers and assistant nurses, with doctors found only at district hospitals. Sometimes a health center will contain a few beds for some maternity cases or emergencies, pending referral to a hospital. The smallest rural facilities are sometimes called rural posts or stations, where a single health auxiliary, with a small supply of government-supplied drugs, lives in a village.

Health centers, staffed by a general practitioner and a pediatrician, along with nurses and others, are the standard facility for ambulatory care in the rural areas of the socialist countries of Eastern Europe. In the main cities, where specialists are found, the ambulatory units are considered polyclinics, although generalists also work in them. It is interesting to note that Great Britain, after great initial resistance to the idea by general practitioners, is now rapidly developing health centers for housing family doctors along with public health nurses and social workers; the general practitioner sees the patients on his panel, for which he is still paid by capitation, rather than being a salaried employee. Such health centers are now being built by local health authorities both in large English and Scottish cities and in small towns. A similar movement is starting in New Zealand, even though the general practitioners under this country's national health service are paid by fee-for-service.

On every continent the concept of an orderly network of facilities is developing, with health centers operating as satellites of hospitals. Patients are sent from the health center to the hospital for diagnostic work-ups and treatment; after hospital discharge, the patient is referred back to the health center for follow-up care. In the Soviet Union, a regular policy of exchange of positions is carried out between health centers and hospitals, for one or two months per year, so that the doctor in each setting can learn about the problems in the other setting. In the United States, the "neighborhood health centers" for the poor have been largely pursued in urban slums, but they probably have important implication for rural areas as well. Private group practice clinics, it may be noted, involve a higher percentage of the total doctors in rural counties than in urban counties, and one can anticipate a wider role for such clinics in the future.

TRANSPORTATION AND COMMUNICATION

A critical aspect of rural health service is the availability of transportation and communication. It is likely that greater benefits have been brought about in rural health care through improved transportation than through enlargement of medical resources in the isolated rural districts.

Most fundamental are paved roads which, of course, serve the general marketing needs of agriculture as well as health services. It is ironic that in various countries of Southeast Asia it took the contingencies of guerilla warfare to produce a network of roads which were long needed anyway for the welfare of rural people; those roads can fortunately facilitate movement of village people to the cities for medical care. On the roads are buses and occasionally taxis for seriously sick patients. Ambulances are also attached to most of the district rural hospitals in Latin America and Asia.

The mobile clinic is widely used in the developing countries as a way of reaching villages distant from a health center. In Malaysia, the Hospital Assistant makes the rounds of several villages once or twice a month, traveling in a small truck that carries a supply of the common drugs. Latin American mobile clinics usually include a doctor along with a nursing assistant. In Africa, rivers are sometimes used as channels for mobile clinics. A certain romanticism attaches to these patterns, but one must realize that a permanent health post, with an auxiliary worker, is nearly always preferable; a medical consultant can then come by periodically.

Home calls by the doctor are becoming rare in most countries, as the demands on the doctor's time have increased. The public health nurse or home visitor is more often sent to investigate matters in rural districts. Yet in Great Britain, the general practitioner is often proud of his continued willingness to make home calls and thereby become acquainted with the real living conditions of his patient. In Belgium, the social insurance program pays the country doctor not only for the mileage involved in home calls, but also for the time consumed in travel, over and above the fee for the medical service.

For extremely isolated rural people, the airplane ambulance is another important adjustment. In Saskatchewan, Canada, when many roads are blocked by snow through the long winter, the airplanes of the provincial Health Department, notified by telephone or radio, pick up patients and transport them to the main cities; many a nighttime landing has been made on a snow-covered wheat field, illuminated by the headlights of three or four automobiles placed to mark out a runway. The stretches of Siberia have long been served also by airplane ambulances, and in Poland helicopters are used. Australia has its Royal Flying Doctor Service—a voluntary agency aided by government grants. More reliance is placed on radio communication and transport of the patient than on conveyance of the doctor. Communication by television is the latest adjustment to rural health care problems; the patient's picture is televised to an urban consultant who then advises a general practitioner out in the field what should be done. This is now being done between Seattle, Washington, and Alaska.

QUALITY PROMOTION AND MAINTENANCE

The isolation of rural health workers makes it difficult for them to keep up with advances in medical science, quite aside from the poverty of rural resources. Everywhere this problem has been tackled through the principle of regionalization, under which small peripheral rural facilities come under the influence of larger urban units.

Regionalization of services is the model for the rural areas of India, Indonesia, Brazil, Sweden, the Soviet Union, mainland China, almost everywhere. The more difficult cases are sent from the peripheral facilities into the central ones, and supervision emanates from the centers outwardly. Rural health personnel may be brought into the main city for various courses of training. Medical schools, of course, along with other types of professional

schools, bear a special responsibility for such continuing education. Sending medical students out to work with rural doctors is
not only valuable for the student but also helps to keep the practitioner on his toes.

In the United States, the regionalization idea got its first major
boost with the Hill-Burton hospital construction program, mentioned above. But it took the Regional Medical Program for
Heart Disease, Cancer, and Stroke to extend the idea to a functional level. Except for the recent major cutbacks in federal RMP
funds, this program was helping to extend the qualitative influence of urban medical centers to rural localities.

ECONOMIC SUPPORT

Basic to the solution of rural health care problems everywhere
is attaining adequate economic support. In many countries, the
social insurance device has strengthened the economic base of
medical care in the cities, where insured wage earners live. But,
most agricultural populations are not brought under the social
insurance or social security umbrella for reasons that are economic,
administrative, and political. As a result, rural health services
have more often depended on support from general national
revenues.

In the Scandinavian countries, district doctors are supported
in the rural areas by the central government, even though they
may also earn fees from the health insurance program. The operating costs of health centers and rural hospitals in the developing
countries are met typically from national revenues. In the United
States, the special comprehensive health care programs for American Indians, a largely rural people, are financed by the federal
government. The same applies to special family health clinics for
migratory or seasonal agricultural workers; formerly all federal,
these are now supported by federal grants to the states. In Yugo-
slavia and Poland, small farmers form health cooperatives for
meeting both construction and operational costs of certain rural
health centers.

As long as the economic base of rural medical care depends
solely on rural people, deficiencies must persist; agriculture simply

has lower per capita productivity than industry with its greater use of machine power and technology. Rural health care can reach the level of urban health care only by tapping urban wealth. In most countries this is done through the use of various types of general revenue. The United States today is debating the issue of national health insurance, as a means of greatly extending economic support for the whole population. We know that voluntary health insurance protection is weakest among rural people, so there is no doubt that rural people would be the greatest beneficiaries of such a nationwide program. With such economic underpinning, one could begin to have hope of getting improvements in the health personnel, facilities, and programs that rural areas need.

HEALTH SERVICE PLANNING AND COORDINATION

The cities, in a sense, can take care of themselves medically, even though there may be extravagance in the use of resources. For improvement in rural health care, planning is always needed at the national or regional level. This has been recognized in India, in almost all the countries of Africa, in most Latin American countries, and throughout the socialist world.

Health planning has come somewhat later to the industrialized countries of Western Europe and North America, where free private enterprise has been so strong. Yet in America today, comprehensive health planning has now been launched in all the states, since the federal grants of 1966 for this purpose. So far, the CHP programs have accomplished little, but we all know that this is because they have no real authority and very little money. The current period, in my view, is a prelude to planning—a tooling-up period. The action will not really begin until we have a program of nationwide economic support for health services, which will provide the resources and, at the same time, the visible urgency to see that the money is wisely spent.

These eight approaches to solving rural health care problems around the world will doubtless sound familiar. There are very few, among the many specific actions, which have not already been tried somewhere in the United States, though not always with adequate intensity. In West Virginia, with its history of health insurance plans in the mining industry (from the old check-off to the modern United Mine Workers of America Trust Fund program), its especially strong program of vocational rehabilitation services, its rural hospital construction program, its impressive new School of Medicine, and its recent legislation on new forms of paramedical personnel, I suspect that the efforts have been more positive than in most states.

The ultimate solution to rural health care problems, however, as one can see everywhere, is not to be found solely within the borders of rural states or provinces. It demands action on a national level both for mobilization of economic support and for allocation of resources in some proportion to need. Along with these moves, which obviously require governmental initiative, people within a state can organize existing manpower and institutions to be better prepared for national developments. Today we see, for example, the clear invitation from Washington to set up "health maintenance organizations" as a sound way to systematize both the financing and delivery of health care. We also see many hints at forthcoming expanded support for training new types of health manpower. These steps will strengthen the groundwork for a national health insurance program, which is sure to come in the new few years. With this, the prospects of improving rural health services should become brighter than ever before.

Chapter 6

THE POTENTIAL ROLE OF THE MEDICAL SCHOOL IN RURAL HEALTH CARE DELIVERY

Leslie A. Falk

These remarks are dedicated to Charlotte, Margaret, and Joseph Yablonsky. Their efforts to improve rural health, as part of a better total life for people in coal mining areas, are well known to many of us. They were murdered in one of many episodes in the brutal sacrifice of human life in the coalfields.

Charlotte graduated in Social Work from West Virginia University and a memorial fund to her is based here. She worked not many miles from here, in and near the Centerville (Pennsylvania) Clinic. Her father and I helped to create this comprehensive care center when he was International Board Member of District 5, United Mine Workers of America, and I was Pittsburgh Area Medical Administrator for the United Mine Workers of America Welfare and Retirement Fund. Fairmont (West Virginia) Clinic is part of those same efforts.

We honor not only them but also those miners and families who are and have been, for democracy. These mountains are a peculiar mix of democracy, racism, and ethnic prejudice. The Manumission Society was advocating the abolition of slavery and publishing the first abolitionist newspaper, *The Emancipator,* in eastern Tennessee in the 1830's and inspiring William Lloyd Garrison to become an abolitionist. The main route from the plantations toward freedom of the Underground Railroad by which slaves escaped bondage before the Civil War ran through the Appalachian mountains and rural communities. These are ample testimony of its historical devotion to freedom.

But is there not also room to suspect that it was easier for the murderers to kill two women and a man with a Slavic name, Yablonsky, when the murder plot was hatched?

It is a pleasure to have the opportunity to participate with such outstanding sponsors and colleagues. Of these, I will name just two. Dr. Milton I. Roemer's book *Rural Health and Medical Care,* co-authored with Dr. Frederick D. Mott in 1948 is still a classic.[1] Two years before that he had written on health in the South.[2] He continues to write illuminatingly on these subjects. Helen Johnston is the second. We have been attending rural health conferences together for over a quarter of a century.

My observations will tend to focus on Appalachia and on the South.

POTENTIAL VERSUS ACTUAL ROLE

The potential role of the medical school in improving rural health care delivery will be stressed here, because most medical schools' actual roles in rural health care delivery leave a great deal to be desired. (The term "medical," as used here, will connote other professions such as nursing, dentistry, and pharmacy.)

Our medical schools have tended to substitute so-called "science" for personal health services, "super-specialization" for continuous unification of health care. They have added to the "brain drain" and, worse, to the "heart drain" from the mountainous and rural areas, tending to convert rural medical students (and their wives) into "big-city folk" or at least institution-focused technologists, whereas rural health care providers and rural community leaders should have been at least one major model.

Schools tend to dissipate the desire of graduates to return to or go to rural areas. Specialists are produced who spend most of their time caring for middle and upper income people. The rural general practitioner is not often relieved by a *locum tenens*, a house-staff doctor, or by others of the health team, nor is he given the stimulation of teaching students.[3]

Medical students tend to acquire more cynicism year by year, much of it due to the signals (overt or subtle) given by their teachers. The humanitarian attitudes measured among first-year medical students become progressively less each year of undergraduate and graduate medical education. There is delaying and even discouragement of a patient-care problem-solving focus in the training of doctors of a primary care relationship.

Are these words too harsh? Of course they are if we take the best examples of the best medical school rural health care programs. For example, the excellent University of Kentucky Community Health Programs and the West Virginia University Medical School has conducted many rural health activities and intends more.

But our United States medical schools have tended to: a) concentrate on patients in hospital beds or in myriads of categorized clinics in complex hospitals; b) exclude the rural family and rural community representatives from the health process; and c) give medical students and housestaff the wrong attitudes toward rural people, especially the poor. The local doctor is "behind the times." The rural folk healer is "superstitious." The emotions-manager, who tends to be the preacher, is "primitive."

THE DOCTOR AND THE HEALTH TEAM

What kind of doctors should the medical schools be preparing? The mission of the doctor in India about 600 B.C. was given as the following:

> To the sick man, the doctor is a father, to the man in health a friend; the sickness past and health returned a preserver.[4]

This definition is near to Dr. Henry Sigerist's 1946 "outlines of a new physician":

> In close touch with the people he disinterestedly serves, a friend and leader, he directs all his efforts toward the prevention of disease and becomes a therapist where prevention has broken down—the social physician protecting the people and guiding them to a healthier and happier life.[5]

The Indian teacher according to the Ayur-Veda should expect the following of a medical student:

> chaste and temperate, to speak the truth, to obey him in all things and to wear a beard.[6]

THE RURAL AND MOUNTAIN COMMUNITY

What rural families are we talking about? Are they mountain people like West Virginians or plainsmen like Kansans; rich rural or poor rural folk; with or without transportation, telephone service, education or money?

To summarize quickly, we know that many rural people tend to be poor, educationally disadvantaged, and caught in demoralizing vicious circles.

In Appalachia, the health problems are numerous. Prematurity, perinatal and infant mortality rates tend to be high, and, as elsewhere, highest among the poor and minority groups. Pregnant women often have protein, mineral, and vitamin malnutrition. Many children have iron deficiency anemia and worms.[7,8] They do not receive immunizations against most preventable diseases.[9] Eye care and dental care are often lacking. The coal miners tend to have "black lung," i.e. coal workers' pneumoconiosis.[10-15] Tuberculosis and histoplasmosis are problems.[16] Mental health services are sparse.

The physical environment is conducive to accidents—in the mines, on the roads, and from farm equipment. Water tends to be contaminated, with acid mine waste or by pathogenic organisms. Housing is substandard in space, in heat control, and in ease of cleaning. The scars of the strip mine and the clutter of abandoned rusting old cars and other old junk defile the natural beauty of the mountains and the once-pure streams.[17]

APPALACHIA'S HEALTH CARE DELIVERY PROBLEMS

On April 20, 1971, a story in *The New York Times* had this to say:

> The poor of Appalachia told a Senate Health subcommittee today that the medical care they received was as deficient as the eroded hollows and strip-mined land in which they lived.
>
> Others told members of the subcommittee, who wandered 100 miles through the northern part of West Virginia, that they were unable to afford medicine.
>
> Mrs. Delores Kemphfer wept as she described the illnesses of the five children she has had in eight years and of the frustrations of obtaining limited medical care because although she and her husband had little money, they were not considered poor enough to get welfare aid.
>
> Ten miles away on a dirt road leading to an abandoned coal mine, Mrs. Edna Moats greeted the Senators from the shambles of her front porch.
>
> Mrs. Moats, who was missing most of her front teeth, was covered with a layer of coal dust, as were several of her six children. She said the nearest water supply was a mile away and water was too precious to use for washing.
>
> A daughter, Helen, played "Silent Night" on a small organ while Mrs. Moats' mentally retarded son, Cecil, played with what looked like part of an automobile transmission in a yard filled with rusty

autos and other junk. Mrs. Moats' husband died eight years ago of black lung disease contracted while working in the coal pits.

Dr. Murray Hunter, medical director of the Fairmont Clinic, Fairmont, West Virginia which the party visited, said health insurance alone would not bring health care to all those who needed it.

Dr. Hunter said the nation's medical care system badly needed reform. Only by reorganizing the services will conditions improve, he said.[18]

HEALTH CARE SYSTEMS IN MINING AREAS

Historical studies of prepaid medical care among iron miners[19] and some other rural prepaid group practices[20] have been conducted by Dr. Jerome Schwartz. The author reviewed United States coal mining health care delivery and payment patterns tracing their British origins.[21] The "check-off" for medical, pharmaceutical and hospital services, the proprietary hospital, and the "company doctor" were characteristic of this system, and examples still persist.

In 1947, 70 per cent of United States coal miners prepaid their medical care, while only a tiny percentage of the entire United States labor force did. The British "pit clubs" and then the "friendly societies," especially the Miners' Permanent Relief Societies, a system of mutual benefit funds, formed the basis of the United States system. In 1869 in the Maryland and Pennsylvania anthracite coalfields we hear of a wage "offtake" or "check-off" for doctor, drug, and hospital services. The company domination of these plans led to widespread dissatisfaction with the "company doctor" plan.

Ross has related the "life style of the coal miner" to the health care delivery system.[22]

In 1949, the UMWA Welfare and Retirement Fund began an extensive general medical care program which later sponsored a network of group health plans,[23] i.e. consumer sponsored prepaid group practice plans and the Appalachian Regional Hospitals health care system.[24]

The state and county health services tend to be understaffed and limited to certain categories; therefore, the mine worker system was necessarily quite comprehensive.

Primary health care is marked by shortages of personnel, and specialists do not abound, but the purchasing power is sizeable. The Hill-Burton hospitals and health department centers have provided many rural communities with adequate regional and district facilities. Regional planning, with improvement of some services, has begun under the Regional Medical Program and the Comprehensive Health Planning Act. State health planning ("A" agencies) have developed under the latter, but at the district level ("B" agencies) relatively little rural progress has been made, primarily for financial reasons, in my opinion.

Important demonstrations exist such as the Frontier Nursing Service of Hyden, Leslie County, Kentucky which has provided nurse-midwife service and now family nurse clinicians, backed by doctors and a hospital.[25] The Appalachian Regional Commission has developed several important health care demonstrations.

Organized home services such as those in the Fairmont (West Virginia) Clinic, the Elkins (West Virginia) Family Health Service and the Appalachian Regional Hospitals are newer unusual examples of nurse and community worker home services, but are limited in the population they can cover.

Nonprofit hospital-based group practice occurs not infrequently. Private medical groups are most common. The Geisinger Memorial Hospital of Danville, Pennsylvania[26] is on the Mayo Clinic fee model. The Appalachian Regional Hospitals recently have tended to assume a regional comprehensive health care model, with outreach and continuity by the personal health team.

Comprehensive health center models, as developed with the Office of Economic Opportunity[27] and the new HEW Section 314 program, reach some rural communities such as the Mountaineer Family Health Plan, Inc. of Beckley, Raleigh County, West Virginia and Lowndes County, Alabama.[28]

The nature of the health team is now fortunately in flux with much needed experimentation. There are examples of primary care (diagnosis, examination, and prescribing treatment) by the new nurse clinician (family health nurse) or nurse practitioner, whatever the new name.[29-30] The physician assistant or MEDEX is also used and production is increasing. "New professional workers" in both the personal and the back-up health team include roles in care analogous to the hospital-based technologist, the office medical assistant, the home, and the community worker.

COMMUNITY PARTICIPATION, CONTROL, OR ADVICE

The place of the community in the health care system has become a matter of activity, discussion, experimentation, and debate, particularly in the United States.[31] The health care provider partnership with the poor has been stimulated by the Office of Economic Opportunity (OEO) health centers,[32] by consumer and trade union leaders in the group health plans, and by politically elected or selected representatives in almost all organized health care developments.

How does all this relate to the medical school?

RESEARCH IN RURAL HEALTH CARE

The medical school is certainly potentially well-equipped to research rural health care delivery and its relation to education. However, this kind of research takes personnel of a kind different from laboratory or clinical investigation. Skills needed include behavioral and social science, health care administration, health economics, systems analysis, computer and communications and community nutrition.

Centers of Health Care Research, financed by the National Center for Health Services and Development, are in a good position to foster this kind of research, but only the barest beginnings have been made. A few examples of subjects requiring or receiving study are the following:

Attitudes and behavior of rural people and of health professionals on the health team. How are the nurse practitioner and physician assistant accepted? What are the health team's actual functions? What district and regional relationships exist?

What are rural peoples' health careers, interests, and educational opportunities?

What patterns seem to attract and, conversely, lose doctors?

What are self-help, health maintenance, and self-care practices in rural communities?

What are local health beliefs? Are there local healers, formal or informal? What do they do?

What are rural life priorities? Where does health care fit in?

In the health care delivery systems, what are the costs and benefits?

Where new comprehensive payment and delivery systems are introduced, does hospital bed use fall or rise?

Are environmental health factors included in the design? What is their place in epidemiological indicators?

Are the occupational health and safety effects and services known?

Can the effect of the health services on outcomes be measured, e.g. on infant mortality and other death rates, on disability, and on morbidity?

MODELS OF ACTUAL MEDICAL SCHOOL RURAL HEALTH CARE DELIVERY

Let us turn now to the medical schools' service relationships to rural health care delivery. Tufts and Rochester, New York, have long had well-developed regional rural relationships, as have many other medical schools.

The American Medical Association's Council on Rural Health describes eleven models for rural health care delivery.[33] Of these, medical schools are described as involved in six. The most common pattern involves medical student participation, sometimes with house-staff, sometimes with nurses. Community-consumer participation tends to another theme.

The University of Kentucky's Frenchburg, Menifer County, Kentucky project was the only one in Appalachia so described in 1969. It has since been discontinued, but other Appalachian medical school plans have come into existence since.

The models described include the following:

Solo Medical Practice of Physicians. A number of medical schools officially sponsor them. Family medicine or general practice preceptorships tend to be the main themes, although specialty rotations of students and residents in community hospitals is another.

Comprehensive Health Care-Community Health Programs. These are illustrated by the University of Florida's program for Fayette County, Florida. In Mayo, sixty miles from Gainesville where the medical school is located, medical residents and several medical students (three or four at a time) provide services in a clinic and at home. They write a health column for a weekly newspaper, teach in the high schools, and appear at church groups. Citizen participation is through a Community Advisory Committee.

Rural Group Practice. The University of Oklahoma Medical Center, through its Department of Preventive Medicine and Community Health, developed a group practice (with faculty appointments for the local doctors) in Waketa, Grant County, Oklahoma. Resident physicians in preventive medicine and in family practice, medical students, and other health care students participate.

Nurse-Focused Primary Care. The University of New Mexico Departments of Pediatrics and of Community Medicine were providing service built around trained nurse-practitioners, especially trained for the responsibilities involved, including public health nurse-midwives. Two half-day visits per week by medical school doctors served this Hope Medical Center in the Estancia Valley, Torrance County, Arizona. Laboratory specimens and x-rays are collected and sent to the Medical Center.

Elective Rural Primary Specialty Service. The Maine Coast Regional Health Facilities Plan, Ellsworth, Maine had Harvard Medical School students on an elective basis in rural pediatrics.

Observation of Private Family Medicine Practice. This was the style of the Iowa College of Medicine—tuition forgiveness for graduates remaining in Iowa, a medical school emphasis on general practice, and "selling of wives" of physicians on the advantages of living in county seat towns were advocated by the state medical society as complementary programs.

The University of Kentucky's rich experiences in rural health have been reported extensively.[34-38] All the medical schools of Appalachia and the South have some aspect of their program which could be described as rural.

MEHARRY AND RURAL HEALTH CARE

What about Meharry Medical College rural experiences? Meharry has had a national and, indeed, international experience in its almost unique role for over ninety-five years in the United States in training black health care professionals. Many rural and mountain area physicians, dentists, nurses, and pharmacists around the world are among its alumni, and many communities look to it for participation in their health care delivery systems. A college-wide program and grant in Community Health Sciences have allowed additional attention to rural health care delivery.[39]

Field faculty members are appointed in various communities. Their school-wide role has consisted primarily of activity in continuing education of physicians. Recently they have tended to become highly involved in health care delivery systems, some of them rural.

The Surgery Department has had a full-blown clinical clerkship for many Meharry Medical students and a surgical residency rotation through the Mound Bayou (Mississippi) Community Hospital ever since 1942. Mound Bayou is over an hour's drive south of Memphis, Tennessee, in Volivar County in the Mississippi Delta country. The medical school service grew out of the needs and abilities of a mutual benefit society with members living primarily in the rural southeast, the Sons and Daughters of Tabor, whose funds enabled them to build the Taborian Hospital which was then staffed through Meharry.

In 1965, Dr. Jack Geiger, then of Tufts Medical School, and Dr. Matthew Walker of Meharry cooperated in obtaining OEO funds to develop the Delta Health Center as a comprehensive community health center, while the Mound Bayou Community Hospital was developed as a teaching hospital and out-patient system.[27]

In addition to in-center services, environmental health services have been given major attention by the Delta Health Center. Indeed, the project director is an environmental health specialist. Home environment has been improved through stimulating new housing and housing rehabilitation. New jobs have been developed. Malnutrition and hunger prevention have been approached boldly by forming a food producing and marketing co-operative, with emphasis on "soul food."

Sunflower County, home of Senator James O. Eastland and of Mrs. Fannie Lou Hamer, is a neighboring county. For two successive summers now, the Department of Family and Community Health of Meharry Medical College has had medical and dental students working on the Sunflower County health care delivery systems. They are assessing its present status and prescribing for it. How can a primary care health center within the county be achieved as the residents want? How can they develop more district interchange with the Bolivar County-Mound Bayou services and with regional resources? Mrs. Hamer serves as a consumer-community field faculty preceptor and cooperates with professional level health care preceptors in working with these students.

The Department of Family and Community Health has a field faculty member in Knoxville, Tennessee. His specialty is preventive medicine and the delivery of health services; his position is Area Medical Administrator, United Mine Workers of America Welfare and Retirement Fund.

Faculty participation has related to mountainous Appalachia as well, e.g. in the Jellico-Model Valley, Tennessee, vicinity. The upper east Tennessee tri-cities vicinity and the Chattanooga-TVA area are also places where the Department has invested time and effort, much of it in cooperation with the Tennessee Mid-South Regional Medical Program and much of this effort within the framework of the Vanderbilt Student Health Coalition, perceptored primarily by Dr. Amos Christie, Emeritus Professor of Pediatrics at Vanderbilt. Its Student Health Coalition utilized the style of Student Health Organization and Student American Medical Association programs, raised monies to support students from other schools as well, developed a year-round activity, and fostered at Vanderbilt what is now a Center for Health Care Delivery.[40]

In southern West Virginia a Meharry field faculty member is an occupational chest disease expert, especially in coal workers' pneumoconiosis ("black lung").

In Lee County, Arkansas, there is a new consumer-poor people sponsored rural health center, located in Marianna, fifty-six miles southwest of Memphis. Independent farmers, tractor drivers on plantations, ministers, insurance men, teachers, housewives, and others have cooperated with VISTA (now ACTION) to found a rural comprehensive care health center. Two Meharry medical students were there for a three-month summer in 1971. The author is on its Board of Directors. The Pine Bluff, Arkansas, and Memphis field faculty members assist it as feasible.

Meharry's Obstetrics and Gynecology Department has a regular residency rotation with Tuskegee, Alabama, the center of Alabama's famous "black-belt counties." Meharry's Pediatrics Department has had a long-continuing tie with Tuskegee Institute and Tuskegee's two teaching hospitals.

FINANCING OF MEDICAL SCHOOL ACTIVITIES IN RURAL HEALTH CARE

Foundation, state, and county monies are sometimes available for these activities. However, like most health expenditures, the Federal Government must play the major role in enabling medical schools to work in rural health care delivery and education in Appalachia and in the South.

The main issue, it seems to me, is the question of special project grants or a unitary national health financing system.

Medicare and Medicaid are, of course, important sources of income, the former on a "rights" basis, the latter on a "means test" basis. Of the new financing sources, the Nixon Administration's backing of Health Maintenance Organizations is a significant 1971 fact.[41] Such support can include some start-up costs for comprehensive care plans, as prepaid group practice or as solo practice, as long as there is a ceiling on expenditures. The benefits must be "comprehensive" enough to include in-patient and out-patient hospital care, medical visits in the office, and home ambulatory laboratory and x-ray services.

National health insurance is in the air. There are basically two different kinds of proposals before the country now. The Administration, the AMA, Representative Fulton and Senator Russell Long would all put more federal dollars essentially into the existing delivery system and into voluntary health insurance channels.

The Health Security Bill of Senators Kennedy, Saxbe, and twenty-four others would finance a unified national health payment system, administered by government agencies, and would allocate much more money to reorganize the delivery system, adding substantial monies for health care education and for developing health care facilities. These would be especially of the consumer-sponsored prepaid group practice variety. Some 5 per cent of the total Federal Health Insurance budget for a Health Security Fund would be so used, in effect.

Which approach would be better for rural areas? An outstanding conceptualization of the standards which legislation should meet was written by the recently deceased Dr. E. R. Weinerman.[42-43] He wrote the following:

> (We need) a program for the production and quality control of manpower and facilities as an essential counterpart to the financing mechanism. It is recommended therefore that a closely coordinated program be established for health resource development and that assured tax support by provided for its adequate financing.

This led to the Health Security Fund in the "Kennedy Bill." Weinerman urged that such a fund regularly assign an appropriate portion of its monies for the following:

> maintenance and improvement of standards of resources, for demonstrations of better methods of training and construction for experimentation with new types of personnel and facilities, and for liaison with other agencies having responsibilities for general educational training of health manpower and for construction of facilities in the health field.

Under the heading "Utilizing the health insurance mechanism as an instrument for reorganization of the service system," he proposed positive incentives toward group practice, but would allow freedom of choice of the following:

> payment on a capitation, salary or fee basis, as elected by the group unit. Since there is adequate evidence that group practice is actually more economical, this would mean higher than average incomes for efficient group practice physicians.

He meant particularly that expensive in-hospital room and board is avoided through comprehensive prepaid group practice, a finding which has been demonstrated repeatedly in recent decades among plans with strong primary and continuing care design.

He advocated full cost reimbursement for the total health team, to support specified kinds of nonmedical personnel, supportive technical resources, and the full costs of regionalization, e.g. communications and transportation costs for the groups' linkages with long-term care facilities, hospital work, and superspecialty resources. In other words, the physicians would not need to sacrifice personal income in order to support the full team and valid supportive services.

Special financial incentives would be provided to encourage the grouping of physicians through initial higher rates of reimbursement to allow development of a group or group health center facilities and to enable training of allied health personnel ("start up costs").

Reimbursement for quality control and improvement mechanisms such as medical audit by medical peers would be financed, so "differential reimbursement might reward achievement in quality, comprehensiveness of care and cost containment."

Preferential reimbursement would be provided for those training schools and programs which emphasize the primary health team in group practice and with regional arrangements. Such financing would also include the costs of continuous in-service training programs in group practices including both work-study programs and refresher continuing education training on a leave basis.

These recommendations were essentially incorporated in S.3, the "Kennedy Bill."

In an intense national development of this kind, predictions are risky. Whatever the developments, however, it seems clear that the medical school and its teaching hospital are, and must be, the regional hub of the system. In turn, involvement of students on a problem-solving basis in rural health care delivery systems seems essential to a sound approach. If this is the case, the medical school must share with the rural community operational responsibility of some kind for such rural health care delivery models. At the very least, it must assure high levels of teaching-learning opportunities with objective evaluations and/or educational research. The rural field faculty method seems one promising method. Through the continuous improvement of such efforts, it is hoped that the potential role of the medical school in rural health care delivery soon becomes its actual role.

REFERENCES

1. Mott, F. D. and Roemer, M. I.: *Rural Health and Medical Care.* New York, McGraw-Hill, 1948.
2. Roemer, M. I.: Present Day Levels of Health in the South. Southern Rural Health Conference, Chattanooga, Tennessee, June, 1946.
3. Sheps, C. G., Wolf, George A., and Jacobsen, C.: Medical education and medical care. Report of a teaching institute. American Association of Medical Colleges. *J Med Ed,* 1961, Part 2.
4. Puschmann, T.: History of Medical Education. (1891) Facsimile reprinted for the New York Academy of Medicine, New York, Hafner Publishing Company, 1966, p. 16.
5. Sigerist, Henry: *The University at the Crossroads.* New York, Schuman Publishers, 1946.
6. Puschmann, T.: *Ibid.,* p. 8.
7. Hutcheson, R. H., Jr.: Iron deficiency anemia in Tennessee among rural poor children. *Public Health Rep, 83:*939-43, November, 1968.
8. Gloor, R. F., Breyley, E. R., and Martinez, I. G.: Hookworm infection in a rural Kentucky county. *Am J Trop Med Hygiene, 19:*1007-9, November, 1970.
9. Martin, D. A., Fleming, S. J., Fleming, T. G., and Scott, D. C.: An evaluation of immunization status of white children in a Kentucky county." *Public Health Rep, 84:*605, July, 1969.
10. Rowntree, G. R.: Coal workers' pneumoconiosis. *J Kentucky State Med Assoc, 68:*97-9, February, 1970.
11. Naeye, R. L. and Laqueur, W. A.: Chronic cor pulmonale: Its pathogenesis in Appalachian bituminuous coal workers." *Arch Pathol, 90:* 487-93, December, 1970.
12. Papers and Proceedings of the National Conference on Medicine and the Federal Coal Mine Health and Safety Act of 1969; Public Law 91-173; June 15-18, 1970, Washington, D. C. The Conference, 1970, pp. 91-236.
13. Kerr, L. E.: Coal mine pneumoconiosis. *Indust Med Surg, 25:*355, 1956.
14. Falk, L. A., Zimmerman, J. P., and Bisdee, C. H.: Stroke among a coal mining population. *Johns Hopkins Med J, 120:*380-392, June, 1967.

15. Steele, H. E.: Negro and white miners under Alabama's pneumoconiosis law. *Indust Med Surg, 383-391*, September, 1962.
16. Bender, T. R., Chick, E.W., and Bauman, D. S.: Inter-Agency Collaboration in screening for tuberculosis and histoplasmosis. *West Virginia Med J, 66:*191-2, June, 1970.
17. Chick, E. W., Jarvis-Eckert, M.A., and Flora, R. E.: Health profiles of three hollows in West Virginia." *West Virginia Med J, 65:*145-52, May, 1969.
18. Poor in Appalachia charge a lack of medical care. *New York Times,* April 20, 1971.
19. Schwartz, Jerome: Prepayment medical clinics of the Mesabi Iron Range 1904-1964. *J History Med Allied Sciences, 22:*139-151, 1967.
20. Schwartz, Jerome: Early history of prepaid medical care plans. *Bull History Med, 39:*450-475, 1965.
21. Falk, L. A.: Coal miners' prepaid medical care in the United States—and some British relationships (1792-1964). *Med Care, 4:*37, 1966.
22. Ross, M. H.: Papers and Proceedings of the National Conference on Medicine and the Federal Coal Mine Health and Safety Act of 1969. *op cit.,* pp. 243-256.
23. Falk, L. A.: Comprehensive care in medical care programs: The U.M.W.A. Welfare Fund. *Med Care, 6:*401-411, September-October, 1968.
24. Falk, L. A.: Group health plans in coal mining communities. *J Health Hum Behav, 4:*4, 1963.
25. Fox, M. P.: Leslie county health program. *Kentucky Med Assoc J, 67:* 504, July 1961.
26. Buchert, W. I.: The Geisinger Story. Hope in the Hills. *Pennsylvania Med, 73:*45-6, July, 1970.
27. Falk, L. A.: The Matthew Walker Health Center of Meharry Medical College Neighborhood Health Center. *Tennessee Med Assoc J, 63:* 849, October, 1970.
28. Hamner, R. T.: Comprehensive health service program in Lowndes County, Alabama. *Med Assoc State of Alabama J, 38:*721-3, February, 1969.
29. Anonymous: A training program for development of the family nurse practitioner. *Frontier Nurses Service Quart Bull, 45:*34-40, Summer, 1969.
30. Borsay, M.: Somer factors involved in the acceptance and rejection of the family nurse. *Frontier Nurses Service Quart Bull, 46:*3-13, Autumn, 1971.
31. Notkin, H. and Notkin, M.S.: Community participation in health services: A review article.*Med Care Rev, 27:*1178-1201, December, 1970.
32. Falk, L. A.: Community participation in the neighborhood health center. *Nat Med Assoc J, 61:*493-497, November, 1969.

33. Health Care Delivery in Rural Areas, Selected Models. Council on Rural Health, American Medical Association, 1969.

34. Deuschle, K. W. and Eberson, F.: Community medicine comes of age. *J Med Educ, 43*:1229-37, December, 1968.

35. Kane, R. L. and Fulmer, H. S.: Residency Training in Community Medicine. A New Concept Utilizing Proven Principles. *Arch Environ Health, 18*:884-7, May, 1969.

36. Steinman, D.: Health in rural poverty: Some lessons in theory and from experience. *Am J Public Health, 60*:1813-23, September 1970.

37. Kane, R. L.: Community Medicine—A perspective for medical students. *Brit J Med Educ, 2*:249-51, December, 1968.

38. Steinman, D. and Deisher, J.P.: SAMA's Summer in Kentucky—Preliminary Evaluation. *Kentucky Med Assoc J, 68*:164-9, March, 1970.

39. Community health sciences teaching grant for Meharry. *Meharry Med Quart Dig*, pp. 3-4, 1971.

40. Spang, Bruce (Ed.): New form of mission in Appalachia. *Vanderbilt Divinity Rev*, Nashville, Tennessee, Spring, 1971.

41. President Nixon's Health Message, The White House, February, 1971.

42. Background Paper for the Committee on National Health Insurance. Available from the CNHI, December, 1969, 27 pp.

43. Falk, L. A.: Functional group practice in a national health program; E. R. Weinerman's last major paper, *Yale J Biol Med*, August, 1971. (in press).

Chapter 7

RELATING PAN-AMERICAN EXPERIENCE TO THE SOLUTION OF RURAL HEALTH PROBLEMS IN THE UNITED STATES

ABRAHAM DROBNY

THE EXPERIENCES in solving the rural health problems in Latin America may or may not be relevant to the health problems in the United States. We will, however, attempt to describe them and to summarize the solutions and approaches, which vary in accordance with the characteristics of each country that have been undertaken by the various governments. At the end we will see which approach or elements of the various methods could be applied to the United States. This undoubtedly is pretentious on our part, since we do not know enough of the health problems in the rural areas of this country except for what we have read in various publications, occasional visits to rural areas, and a very enlightening trip to some counties in West Virginia at the kind invitation of Dr. Robert Nolan.

The first problem in the approach to the so-called rural areas in Latin America and the Caribbean is to reach a working definition of "rural area," since there are countless variables to be considered. The definition varies according to the developmental characteristics of each country. Most counties express it in terms of numbers of inhabitants, and that number varies from 1,000 to 5,000. The United States, for instance, defines as the rural unit, for census purposes, any township of less than 2,500 inhabitants, though Professor Wilson G. Smillie stated that for the purposes of public health administration a suitable rural unit of population is from 25,000 to 50,000 or more people.

There are countries that give a less precise notion of what they consider rural; some of them regard only the capital of the country and the most important towns as urban areas. Others consider all places possessing certain facilities such as water supplies, sewage disposals, or electric power as urban townships, leaving all those without these services as rural. In any case, even though the definition generally accepted is in numerical terms particularly useful for statistical purposes, it is recognized that care must be taken in using it, since no arbitrary classification based on numbers of population can be entirely satisfactory.

RURAL HEALTH SITUATION IN LATIN AMERICA

In the Latin American countries and in the English-speaking Caribbean, rural communities are spread over vast regions where, as a rule, the population is engaged in agricultural work. Without discussing at length the general conditions in the rural areas, let us just say that facilities are quite inadequate. Economic and social problems, which have become chronic in some countries and have led to mass migration into the cities, have created what has been described as "the ruralization of the urban environment."

Distribution of Population

The distribution of urban and rural population in the Americas is rapidly changing. The population of rural areas in twenty-four countries in the Americas in 1967 was over 114 million inhabitants or 47.6 per cent of the total population of those countries. This percentage varies from country to country with a range of 18 per cent in one to 83 per cent in another.

Health Problems

Inadequate reporting of diseases and a general lack of vital and health statistics in the rural areas make it impossible to obtain any exact knowledge concerning the health problems of the rural environment. It may also be pointed out that a high proportion of deaths occurring in rural areas is not medically certified, which makes it difficult to use specific mortality rates to study the scope of the health problems in these areas.

Nevertheless, if we analyze the figures for deaths due to various causes in urban and rural areas, we find a great difference between these two population groups. There are several studies in various countries that compare the general mortality and child mortality rates (both infant and preschool) in predominantly rural zones with those of large urban areas in the same countries. Infant mortality is sometimes two to four times higher in the rural areas.

From the scanty data available, it is also clear that protein calorie malnutrition is a much more serious problem in the rural environment than in the cities. Data are available from studies undertaken in several countries.

Communicable diseases such as malaria, tuberculosis, tetanus, leprosy, Chagas' disease, parasitosis and many others are prevalent in most of the rural areas throughout the continent. Studies by Baldó and Curiel in Venezuela,[2] Villas-Boas in Brazil,[3] and Alvarado, Guzmán and Buroncle in Honduras[4] show a much higher incidence of tuberculosis, for example, in the rural areas than in the urban areas of the same countries. The same could be said for parasitic diseases from studies made by Daensvang in Puerto Rico[5] and the Ministry of Health of Brazil.[6] We could go on with other kinds of studies, as for example, the one made by the Ministry of Health of Venezuela on Chagas' disease[7] and many others which show quite clearly, even though the figures are not reliable enough, that these kinds of problems are clearly more prevalent among rural populations.

The shortage and poor quality of mother and child services aggravate the situation and increase the morbidity and mortality among mothers and children, especially during the first year of life. There is a considerable difference between the infant mortality rates in urban and rural areas, even though in many countries this is not reflected in the official statistics because of lack of proper registration.

There is probably no single factor that has a greater effect on the health, well-being, and development of a community than the provision of an ample and convenient supply of good quality water.

In towns and cities the water supply is recognized as an essential service, a basic necessity for industrial and commercial processes, vital for the maintenance of public health and the prevention of epidemics; without it, many activities are impossible. In rural areas the need is equally great, though usually less well recognized. It is significant that at the 1969 World Health Assembly the delegate from one government in Asia estimated that water borne diseases accounted for 40 per cent of all mortality and 60 per cent of all morbidity in that country.

Since the beginning of 1961, considerable efforts have been made in Latin America to reach the target set by the Charter of Punta del Este, namely, to provide drinking water for 50 per cent of the rural population. In spite of all efforts, the majority of the countries are a long way from achieving this target. As of the end of 1970, 18 per cent of the rural population had either house connection to main water supplies or easy access to them. This figure includes twenty-six countries in Latin America and the Caribbean and the Eastern Caribbean Islands. The range goes from 2 per cent in one country to 91 per cent in another. The 18 per cent compares to 75 per cent as an average for the urban population in the same countries.[8] Even more serious than the situation regarding drinking water is that of excreta disposal; here little has been done up to the present, except sporadic activities in certain countries. The problem of rural sanitation has its direct implication in the diarrheal diseases, all of which are aggravated by the fact that they affect the population group suffering from severe nutritional deficiencies.

Resources for Health Care

Naturally, health services in the rural areas cannot be self-sustained and autonomous. The tendency is to organize them as part of a regional health service system, in which the urban, suburban, and rural areas are suitably combined into self-sufficient regions; thus, in general, rural health care is based on a network of institutions in the various towns of the area, these in turn having subsidiary services for suburban areas and rural health care centers. Ideally all this constitutes a system of a two-way avenue spread over the whole of each country and defined to cover the entire population of the national territory. Most of the Latin American countries, however, are still a long way from attaining this ideal coverage, and there are large numbers of rural communities without even the most rudimentary health service.

To give an idea of the resources, we will mention availability of hospital beds in capitals and large cities as compared to the rest of the countries. For instance, Costa Rica has 6.9 hospital beds per thousand inhabitants in the capital and the large cities, as compared to 2.3 in the rest of the country. The figures for Ecuador are 3.7 and 1.7, respectively. In El Salvador, the figures are 10.7 and 1.1. Guatemala shows figures of 9.9 for the large cities and 1.3 for the rest, Peru's figures are 5.6 and 1.7, Trinidad and Tobago 18.7 and 3.8, and Venezuela 4.6 and 2.9, respectively.[9]

Of course, it should be borne in mind that the information given for the so-called "rest of the country" involves smaller cities and not necessarily rural areas. Unfortunately, we do not have precise information for rural areas, but we can anticipate that the rates would be much lower than those given for the "rest of the country" in each of the cases presented.

If we look at the availability of human resources, we find again an uneven distribution of physicians and other health workers between the large cities and the rest of the areas in each country. I shall give only some of these figures for 1968. Argentina had 33.7 doctors per 10,000 in the capital and large cities compared to 12.1 in the rest of the country. In Barbados the situation was 9.4 for large cities and 1.7 for the rest. Costa Rica showed rates of 12.4 and 3.3, El Salvador 13.9 and 0.6, Chile's rates were 10.3 and 3.3, Mexico 22.9 and 3.0, and Panama had 12.1 physicians per 10,000 in large cities and 2.1 in the rest of the country. This is just to mention some of them. Here again what is considered "rest of the country" is not necessarily the rural situation which one might infer is much worse off. The figures given for physicians also apply to nurses and other health workers.[10]

METHODS UTILIZED TO PROVIDE HEALTH SERVICES FOR RURAL AREAS

Countries have resorted to a variety of schemes in an attempt to provide health services for the rural population. In the main, these services start out from one basic fact common to all of them —that access to the rural environment is difficult, and the rural areas, therefore, are isolated. The difficulty of finding medical practitioners and other professional workers willing to work in these areas has everywhere tended to point in one particular direction, namely, the use of a special type of *ad hoc* personnel, in Latin America, the auxiliary health worker. However, since the characteristics of rural areas are not the same in all countries, and sometimes differ in the different regions of the same country, it has not been possible to establish methods which necessarily apply to all of them. The general trend is to establish a health service infrastructure where none exists, so as to provide rural communities with minimum health care. This infrastructure in most Latin American countries is part of a regional health service system, with a direct line of communication to the next step, which may be a suburban, and above that, a more complete urban health service.

Here we will attempt to analyze briefly only some of the most successful systems being used, or at present being developed, to provide health services for the rural communities.

Early in the 1960's an attempt was made in Venezuela to utilize an assistant physician, similar to the "feldsher" of the Soviet Union, a professional duly trained to diagnose and treat the most frequent and most easily recognizable diseases. This was not accepted by the medical profession. However, a compromise was reached in using nonprofessional trained health auxiliaries within a system that insures proper supervision and referral to higher echelons.

The Venezuelan experience is based on what we have mentioned before, a regionalized health system. The country is thus divided into health regions. In the most important city of each of these regions, complete health services are available including hospital beds with specialized services. Each region has several health districts headed by a Health Center which serves the community by rendering both preventive and curative services. The Health Center is mainly an ambulatory service; however, each one has a certain number of beds, some of them up to 60, which are used for maternity cases and for emergencies. All other cases are transferred to the general hospital.

As a dependent of the Health Center and under its supervision there are several, sometimes eight to ten, so-called *Medicaturas*

Rurales. These are subcenters in populations of two to five thousand inhabitants directed by a full-time general practitioner with special post-graduate training and in permanent contact both through communications and visits with the health center.

The communities below 2,000, which go down to 200 inhabitants, are covered by the so-called *Dispensarios Rurales* which are cared for by the nonprofessional auxiliary that we have mentioned above. Three, four, or five of these auxiliaries are under the responsibility of each Medicatura Rural.

The health auxiliaries are usually selected from the area in which they are going to work. They are given a three-month intensive course by specially trained nurses. These courses are given to a group of around twelve to twenty auxiliaries. After they finish their course they receive a manual which gives them detailed information of what they can do, and especially on what they should not do. The manual or handbook is complete with pictures and figures to give them a graphic view of the various problems with which they are going to work. The auxiliaries' main activities are gathering health statistics and information, preventive activities, and first aid. In practical terms they know exactly what to do when a child comes in with a mild temperature and diarrhea, when they can begin treatment by themselves and when they should refer the patient immediately to the physician of the *Medicatura Rural.* It must be borne in mind that these workers do not replace the nurse or the physician; they are just an addition to the health system in areas where there was no service at all. These auxiliaries are supervised by the physician of the *Medicatura Rural,* the public health nurse, and the sanitarian, in a periodic way so as to have at least one of these health workers visiting every week. They perform vaccinations, including BCG, smallpox, DPT, polio, yellow fever, typhoid, measles, and others. As mentioned before, they give first aid in case of accidents and illnesses in accordance with the instructions in their handbook. They also give advice to the population on simple health education measures and they are trained to advise in the construction of latrines and on garbage disposal. They are not trained in midwifery; however, they do give some prenatal care and refer the patient to the physician when necessary and for delivery.

Another system of providing health care to rural communities which is found in several countries is the one developed by Costa Rica. The Ministry of Health has a network of health units, in total eighty-two of them, located in cities rendering mostly ambulatory services. Some of them have up to 15 maternity beds to take care of normal deliveries. Sixteen of these centers have mobile units to extend their services to more isolated areas. These units are staffed by a recently graduated physician who works full time, an auxiliary nurse specially trained for the purpose, a sanitary inspector, and a driver who also acts as an auxiliary in handling audiovisual equipment for health education purposes. These mobile units visit the rural communities twice per month as an average. They devote their time to community organization, health education, medical care, immunization, and environmental sanitation activities. Mobile services are rendered until a permanent structure is established by the Ministry of Health.

This type of mobile services is limited in certain countries because of its high maintenance costs and because the roads, where available, are not always usable all year around.

Several countries like Ecuador, Colombia, Peru, and others have laws that require that graduate physicians must serve at least one year in a rural community in order to be able to practice. In some other countries, this is done as a rural internship prior to graduation.

Countries like Colombia and Panama also utilize voluntary personnel in accordance with the services they are going to render. However, most of these voluntary workers serve in only a limited capacity, particularly in organizing the rural dwellers in self-help projects, practicing certain vaccinations under instructions of a physician, helping with advice on health education, and related matters.

In the Amazon areas of Peru, where the population is widely scattered and distances are so great that there is little possibility of supervision, school teachers are being used to render first aid and elementary health services. They are given a short period of training and their duties are explained specifically in a handbook, which is both a set of rules and an educational manual. It does not go beyond first aid and very simple treatment for illnesses which are easily diagnosed and do not involve any risk. These school teachers carry out the services without any additional remuneration.

In one country, regions remote from urban centers and having scattered rural populations have been provided with first aid posts operated by the police force. For this purpose the police receive special training. Over a hundred such posts have been set up in Chile in the mountainous region.

In summary, serious deficiencies are still found in most Latin American countries in relation to health care of the rural population. Neither the number of hospital beds nor the network of health centers or rural posts can pretend to cover the needs of the rural population and there are vast zones where no services whatever exist. The same is true as to human resources—there is a marked tendency for both doctors and other professional health workers to concentrate in towns and large cities.

APPLICATION OF THE LATIN AMERICAN EXPERIENCE TO THE UNITED STATES

The situation in many of the rural areas in the United States, if not similar to the one I have described in Latin America, has some common elements. Most of this population is scattered and live in relatively isolated conditions. The topographical characteristics of the rural areas in West Virginia that I have been privileged to visit contribute to the physical isolation, the difficulties in communication, and the inaccessibility to health services. Another common characteristic is the lack of doctors and other health personnel. The few physicians that work in these areas as private practitioners are overworked and the programs of the health departments are very limited and rarely able to make a significant impact upon unmet individual health needs.

The environmental problems, if not the same, have similar characteristics. A good number of homes do not have adequate water and sewage services essential for health. To add to the problems of the rural dweller, no adequate public transportation is available.

All this brings about necessarily higher morbidity and mortality rates than those of the urban communities of the United States.

Here I must point out one main difference in the situation in the Latin American countries as compared to the United States. In Latin America, health care, including preventive and curative services as well as rehabilitation, is provided by Ministries of Health and in some cases Social Security Institutions—private practice being limited to those who can afford it and do not want to make use of the services offered by government. In the United States, cities, counties, and states offer mostly preventive services, leaving medical care as a private endeavor. We do know that states and local governments provide services to indigents; however, these are limited and done mostly through private physicians and hospitals. This fact makes it more difficult to apply to the United States situation any of the Latin American systems to provide rural communities with health services.

One of the aspects of the complex problem of providing health care to rural populations, which is strikingly similar in the United States to the experience in Latin America, is undoubtedly the lack of human resources. For obvious reasons the physician is not tempted to work in this environment. The states and counties either do not have the funds or do not have the interest to provide health services in quality and quantity as needed. Another important point is that sanitation, particularly provision of potable water and sewage disposal, as well as garbage collection or treatment, is lacking in spite of the enormous technological development of the United States. This is undoubtedly not due to lack of know-how to solve the problem, but to some other reasons which are beyond my competence to analyze, as a health worker.

The lack of human resources points out, as it did in Latin America, the need of utilizing paramedical personnel and perhaps even auxiliary personnel—not to replace physicians or nurses, but to given some services where none exist.

Increasing awareness of the inability of existing health manpower to meet growing demands for services has prompted the medical community in several parts of this country to seek innovative ways for increasing the physician's productivity and for expanding his capacity to deliver health care. One method, commanding increasing interest and attention, deals with changing patterns of delegation of selected duties and functions traditionally performed by the physician. Over the past years a variety of experimental programs has come into being in medical centers scattered across the nation. As far as I know no centralization of effort has emerged as yet; there is no standardization of program design or curriculum content, or even certification procedures.

There are a variety of names used to identify a new assistant to the physician which some call "physician's assistant," "clinical associate," "nurse physician associate," "MEDEX," and others.

The former Assistant Secretary for Health and Scientific Affairs of the Department of Health, Education and Welfare, Dr. Roger O. Egeberg announced some time ago the establishment of a national program administrative office for Operation MEDIHC (Military Experience Directed Into Health Careers). He said "This is the first in a series of steps which will be taken to expand significantly the MEDIHC program nationwide." This consists in a counseling and recruiting program for Vietnam and other returning veterans who have health occupation skills, training, and experience. Through MEDIHC, this personnel, with an interest in health careers, may locate civilian employment and training opportunities in the health field prior to being separated from the Armed Forces. In making this announcement, Dr. Egeberg said, "Less than a year ago we initiated Operation MEDIHC in cooperation with the Department of Defense. Today, about 6,500 ex-military corpsmen have received assistance from MEDIHC coordinators in forty-seven states, the District of Columbia, Puerto Rico, and the Virgin Islands. They have been advised about health occupations, training programs, and employment opportunities throughout the country. They are enrolled in junior colleges, colleges, and universities where they are preparing for health careers. They are employed in hospitals, physicians' offices, State and Local Health Departments and other health facilities. These veterans are contributing valuable talents towards meeting the nation's need for more health manpower."[11]

I am sure that the MEDEX program developed at the University of Washington in Seattle is well known to you. This program is creating a new class of medical professionals who are helping overworked physicians provide more and better medical care. I am not going to get into details of this project but would like to emphasize that some of the MEDEX personnel are already working in rural communities of the state of Washington, such as the towns of Tonasket with a population of 1,000 and a smaller town called Twisp with a population of 750. Other MEDEX programs have now been started, one at the University of North Dakota School of Medicine, which has MEDEX personnel in North Dakota, South Dakota, and northern Minnesota.

The Director of the MEDEX program in Seattle, Washington, Dr. Richard A. Smith has reported that there are already over eighteen MEDEX working in eleven states and he feels that there will be approximately 130 in the field in fifteen states by the end of 1971.

This kind of health personnel could very well be used in providing services to rural dwellers. In any case, if the Latin American experience is to be applied to the United States situation, we feel that regionalized health services could be developed, preferably on a statewide basis. If this is not possible, it could be done on a county basis or as a demonstration area using a university medical center as the base of operation, with the aim of both demonstrating what can be done and for training of students of health sciences, with the hope that it would have a multiplying effect in other rural areas.

In referring to the regionalization system, we mean that the base center should be a general hospital with smaller hospitals at an intermediate level, and health centers providing services as close to the rural communities as possible. A good transportation service should be available to refer patients to the higher levels. For the services rendered at the local level the aforementioned new type of professionals could be used, or nurses, or even auxiliary personnel provided they are trained to give first aid, to vaccinate, to educate, and to screen patients that should be referred to the hospital, either at the intermediate or at the central level.

A team formed by a physician, a nurse, and a sanitarian would visit the rural outposts on a periodic basis to supervise, give in-service training, and provide the health care that may be required.

One of the most important aspects of providing services to the rural community is educating the population in joining their efforts to improve the economic and social, as well as, general conditions of the communities. In our experience public health services often serve as the initiators of this process of community development. Another important aspect in the United States situation is that efforts should be made to better utilize institutions and laws already in existence, and usually working in a parallel way, to try to bring about a real coordination and unity of effort.

The sanitarian and, if available, the health educator are of great importance in this activity, particularly in trying to enlist the community in a self-help type of program directed towards sanitation, which can be done through well-digging, latrine construction, or other types of solutions depending on the characteristics of the area.

Even considering that medical care is mostly a private activity in this country, we believe that a system of developing health services can be achieved if not always through the State or County Health Departments, it may be possible to obtain grants from the Federal Government to establish and operate a demonstration area as we have mentioned above.

I do not believe that this will be easy, but the very urgent need and the awareness by many health authorities in this country of the existing problems make me look at it from the optimistic side.

REFERENCES

1. Smillie, Wilson G.: *Preventive Medicine and Public Health*. New York, MacMillan Co., 1949.
2. Baldo, J. I., Curiel, J., and Lobo Castellano, O.: La Tuberculosis Rural en Venezuela. *Boletin of the Pan American Sanitary Bureau,* January, 1965.
3. Villas-Boas, A.: A Tuberculose no Interior de Brasil. *Rev Serv Nac Tuberculose, 10:*38, Rio de Janeiro, Brasil.
4. Alvarado, Guzman A. and Buroncle, A.: Lucha Antituberculosa en el Area Rural de Honduras. *Rev Med Hond, 32,* Tegucigalpa, 1964.

5. Daensvang, S.: *Puerto Rico Journal of Public Health and Tropical Medicine, 7:*359, San Juan, 1936.

6. Distribucao de Esquistosomase Mansonica no Brasil. Ministry of Education and Health, Rio de Janeiro, Brasil, 1950.

7. Campana contra la Enfermedad de Chagas. mimeograph. Ministerio de Sanidad y Asistencia Social, Caracas, 1966.

8. Water Supply. Pan American Health Organization, 1971. mimeograph.

9. Health Conditions in the Americas. Pan American Health Organization Scientific Publication No. 207, September 1970.

10. Health Conditions in the Americas. *Ibid.*

11. Operation MEDIHC. *Milit Med, 523:*136-5, May, 1971.

Chapter 8

MODEL HEALTH CARE DELIVERY SYSTEMS

Murray B. Hunter

I SHALL TRY TO DESCRIBE what we do now at Fairmont (West Virginia) Clinic and its satellite officers—not necessarily as a static model, but as a reasonably durable experiment in providing comprehensive health services to rural and semirural people under the sponsorship of group practice.

Fairmont is the county seat of Marion County which, in common with most West Virginia counties, is experiencing chronic depletion of primary physicians, especially in its outlying towns. Fairmont Clinic was established thirteen years ago as a joint venture. The essential ingredients that secured the traumatic but ultimately successful delivery of this creature were organizations committed to its financial support, the United Mine Workers of America Welfare and Retirement Fund; a body of leading citizens organized as a nonprofit development and property holding corporation, the Monongahela Valley Association of Health Centers; and a pioneer medical staff. From its very outset, it was the policy of the Fairmont Clinic and its sponsors to operate satellite offices. The locations of these dictated primarily by the needs of coal mining families who had lost, through attrition and aging, physicians traditionally resident in their communities. There were originally three such community branch clinics. At present there are two. They replace previous "check-off" arrangements, and for a time certain by-products of check-off arrangements were perpetuated into a new pattern of delivery care, such as medical care grievance committees with direct confrontation of the complaining patient with the alleged offending physician, and stipulated rights to certain medication and to housecalls. The quality and tone of the clinic's subsequent relationship with its main body of constituents, the coal miners, were forged in the process

110

of adaptation from previous check-off arrangements to more "modern" modes.

The branch clinic is totally a part of the central clinic operation at all levels. Hiring of personnel, provision of supplies, payment of rent, maintenance, and other supporting services are all provided by the central clinic. The employees of the branch clinic belong to the same collective bargaining unit as do those at the central clinic. The physicians who staff the branch clinics are full-time members of the Fairmont Medical Group, several of whom have served on its leading committees. They are salaried and their salaries are computed on the same basis of training and experience as those of the physicians working in the central clinic. Identical standards of income determination, hours of work, pension, and other fringe arrangements apply to them as to physicians working in the center. The branch clinics have had a variety of staffing arrangements. Each is staffed by one full-time general practitioner, assisted by a varying array of specialist physician visits from the central clinic. Each branch clinic has regular medical consultation; one has regular pediatric consultation. Both have had surgery and obstetrics/gynecology consultation. The branch clinics do have "health center" functions, in that physical therapy, social work, and home health services have consistently been available in them. They have served the community as a local contact point for vocational rehabilitation services, alcohol information service, and for other *ad hoc* public health functions. Each office has a clinical laboratory and one has an x-ray department. Film is read by the clinic radiologist, a typed report of the reading appended to the chart, and the original film is retained in the branch clinic office.

All records are dictated. The tapes and belts of dictation are picked up daily, typed in the central facility, and the dictation returned to the branch office. Pharmacy services are similarly provided to the branch clinics. There is prescription pick-up daily and drug delivery under extremely controlled conditions.

The physicians who are at the branch clinics participate in the life of the group, attend all of its meetings including its weakly two-hour clinical conference, are members of the single hospital staff to which all group physicians belong, assist in surgery, and admit patients of their own to their own service or to the service of other clinic physicians in the appropriate specialty.

The Fairmont Clinic never insisted that physicians who practice in these communities reside there but it was favored, and for physicians who did reside in the community in which they practiced, a bonus was paid. In salaried group practice a bonus is designed to soothe the pangs of inequitable labor. It was felt that residence in the community of practice could serve to deprive the branch office physician of some of his scheduled share of organized time off. A physician in a small town cannot take his youngster to the ten cent store on his day off and not practice medicine at the same time. Likewise his nights off tend to be less secure. At present no physicians reside in the communities of their branch offices, and night, weekend and holiday coverage is provided for the patients of the branch office out of the central clinic.

A few West Virginia University students have had elective experience in these branch offices.

We have organized no patient transport from the periphery to the center, no electronic hookups, and no closed circuit television. When the branch clinic physician was away on vacation or study time, we provided these offices with medical coverage. However, now the chief nurse at each location functions as a nurse practitioner during vacations without a doctor present, but with considerable back-up from the central clinic; we have had no discernible patient complaint nor adverse turn in quality as a result.

The chief operational difficulty encountered in day-to-day function of the branch clinics is one of poor transfer of information from one center to another on patients whose care is complicated and whose management is shored between the community offices and the central clinic.

It is obvious at this point, in reflecting upon this experience, that the basic model here is the traditional one-to-one doctor-patient encounter. These clinics do have health center trappings (social work, physical therapy, pharmacy service, ancillary support, visiting specialists) but the patient expectation is to get an appointment, see the doctor, and in an emergency come without prior arrangement for service and receive the same.

The question has often been asked within and without our own organization whether this form of rural and semi-rural health care delivery is economical. It has been suggested that the general physician be taken out of primary service and the nurse-practitioner or physician-assistant or other new middle category of health personnel be substituted. In our view, only in the hopefully soon-to-be antiquated fee for service method of cost accounting can such utilization of physician time be regarded as uneconomical. The offices are attractive, facilities are ample, and each full-time physician in the branch clinic is responsible for between 5,000 and 7,000 separate office encounters annually. We are reluctant to part with this in favor of untried newer experimental models, particularly when our experience teaches us that important human values are served by maintaining primary medical facilities as close to peoples' residences as is logistically possible.

Of course, there is no reason that rural health center developments of the type described need a central base of physician practice such as Fairmont Clinic for their support and survival. The unique experience of the Hygeia Foundation in southern West Virginia attests to the fact that widely dispersed centers of care may be kept to standards not only of the amenities of practice but of quality, provided that the financial support and community initiative for facilities development and maintenance is present. In that instance, the visiting specialists are recruited by the board on a part-time basis and do not necessarily have a group relationship among themselves.

Our kind of tight integration of the outlying satellite with the central clinic is both feasible and desirable, given the local topography, up to a radius of about thirty miles from the center. The physicians can practice in the same hospital, patients can travel easily within a half day for consultative services, the physicians can get to know one another and cover one another in times of absence. However, the relationship between large group practices in county seats and small cities and towns ought now to be, of necessity, confined to such tightly constructed norms. One can conceive of many types of arrangements between central group practices and outlying solo or small partnership practices that are not nearly so closely integrated. While we regard other than salaried arrangements as inconsistent with sound principles of group practice, we are not such purists that we would reject a variety of partial relationships with physicians in fee practice or combination arrangements who are in more remote rural settings and who desire supportive relationships with us. Those supportive relationships might be negotiated with physicians already in practice or with community sponsors attempting to structure such relationships in advance of physician recruitment. These supportive relationships might include only home health service, only pharmacy service, only laboratory service, only transport to a diagnostic center, only business office assistance, only physician consultative relationships, only attendance at conference as a "keep-up" service, or any combination of the above. Under such arrangements, the central office clinic may provide the traditionally entrepreneurial solo physician in a remote setting a route out of isolation but not necessarily toward the conformities of group practice.

There is no reason that, in the future, especially under the stimulus of a national health insurance act (whose purpose it would be to guarantee medical care to Americans, not to equalize the odds of getting it) other forms of support and sponsorship for a variety of rural practice models would not be devised. The Regional Medical Program, recently described in a national article as "in search of a mission," might well be a vehicle for sponsoring supportive services to rural practitioners and even encouraging salaried guarantees for them in association with community sponsors. My reasons for caution and a modicum of skepticism flow out of a deep appreciation of the difficulties of group practice maintenance and development, to say nothing of an awareness that in spite of its apparent national popularity, concrete group practice development will continue to meet opposition by local vested elites, even under National Health Insurance. I would like to offer some political advice to rural people. If, under any statute, the Federal Government is to underwrite some or all of the costs of group practice start-up, rural people should insist to the Congress that any proposed new Health Maintenance Organization, certified under new legislation, must, as a condition of certification, undertake a stipulated obligation to redress a maldistribution of medical services. This obligation could apply to the care of a segment of an adjacent inner-city ghetto or an adjacent underserviced rural area. In either instance, however, as a condition of certification, the HMO ought to be compelled to assume its share of responsibility for reversing the present trend toward the rich getting richer and the poor getting poorer with respect to the availability of medical service. It is time that Federal monies were used to create social change rather than, as under Medicare, buttress existing ways of doing things.

I have not made mention of medical schools as co-sponsors of new approaches to rural health care. There is little doubt that there are many schools which have manifested sincere desires in this area and in some, a considerable record of achievement has been written. However, for the most part, the record is poor. Medical education is too often loaded with subtle and not so subtle cues that are antithetical to good practice models. The fact that community or rural clinic practice models are elective rather than required courses in most curricula, perhaps available if the student is interested but hardly on a par with other subject matter, is proof enough that such cues are strongly institutionalized. When the schools demonstrate humanizing values in their own out-patient departments, they conceiveably can seriously undertake the role of more durable long-term responsibility to the health needs of a fixed component of the rural population. In making these remarks let it be understood that I refer to no particular school. We do ask that students be exposed to the many superb models that exist in this state and in Appalachia in general. It is upon the basis of these experiments that new departures in the delivery of health care to isolated populations can be made. We do need help in the form of rational federal legislation in which logic shall reign rather than vested interest. New legislation should interfere with medical practice and should not underwrite the status quo. There are too many counties in this area where medical resources are meager or absent and in them whole new categories of care and types of plans for care will have to be created. We neither need nor want, on a national level, a pretense of planning for nonexistent resources to provide nonexistent services. A definite time should be set, as in the proposed

Viet Nam pull-out, at the end of which every American shall be guaranteed the availablity of modern medical care. Between the pasage of new law and the introdutcion of that new medical care system, every effort should be bent to the development of new resources and their locations in places of need.

Chapter 9

THE FAMILY NURSE AND PRIMARY HEALTH CARE IN RURAL AREAS

Gertrude Isaacs

T HE FAMILY NURSE as a provider of primary health care is a relatively new concept in this country. The nurse has, however, been used in this capacity by the Frontier Nursing Service (FNS) for forty-six years. The FNS is a comprehensive primary health care service and training center located in the Appalachian region of southeastern Kentucky. It provides services in Leslie County and parts of Perry and Clay. The program is currently being extended because of the continuing shortage of medical manpower in rural areas and the growing demand for improved health services. The family nurse who forms the nucleus of the service is a registered nurse with special preparation in the health field.

The Frontier Nursing Service was developed to meet the crucial needs of rural areas in 1925. The health manpower crisis is not new to the rural areas; it is only the social cognition which is new. Individuals like Mary Breckinridge recognized it much earlier. Her aim was to develop a system whereby health services could be made accessible to the people at a price they could afford. The nurse-midwife was selected at the outset to provide the primary health services. After forty-six years of experience, she continues to be the basic professional for many reasons.

1. The nurse-midwife has many of the basic skills needed to provide family services, and given additional training in diagnosis and management of common health problems, she can readily extend her services to the total family.

2. The use of the family nurse helps lessen manpower problems in rural areas. There are two to three nurses to every physician in this country, and nurses are geographically

117

more equitably distributed than the physician. This helps reduce the recruitment problem.

3. In one year a nurse can be prepared to provide primary health care. Therefore, care can be provided at a lesser cost and more accessible to the people.

4. By using the nurse in this capacity, the physician is freed to use his skill to better advantage, and overall health care can be markedly improved.

5. Traditionally the nurse has been trained to be more involved in helping the family cope with the day-to-day problems of health and illness, primarily a nurturant role. The physician, on the other hand, has been much more involved in the intricacies of diagnosis and treatment of disease—a curative role. Both are of vital importance in health service. In underdeveloped areas, however, the nurturant role is of particular importance because people in these areas are less well prepared to deal with the problems of health and illness. The physician tends to get bored with these problems, while nurses continue to accept this aspect of care as a challenge. The nurse for these reasons is particularly well suited for this role.

Both the role of the nurse and the system in which she operates are unique. The system is designed to reach out to the people; and as stated earlier, the nurse rather than the physician forms the nucleus of the service. Instead of a big central station with all the latest modern equipment and specialty services to which patients may have to travel long distances to receive health care, the Frontier Nursing Service has a series of very moderately equipped nursing outposts in the communities where the people live. These outposts are strategically situated. No family living in a nursing district is further than one hour's travel time from a primary health center. Each outpost, in turn, has ready access to the hospital and health center where a resident physician is available at all times. He may, if necessary, refer the patient to specialty services outside the area. For example, a patient may be referred to or consultation sought from one of the nearby regional hospitals or the University of Kentucky Medical Center, depending on his need. This network makes it possible to provide the best of medical care available in the state to the most isolated patient in the area. It also helps keep primary health care more personalized.

The Frontier Nursing Service has a total of approximately 53,000 out-patient contacts a year. The majority of the patient contacts, approximately 30,000, occur at the nursing outposts. Each outpost is staffed by one or two nurses, and a single nurse serves an average population group of 200 to 250 families or 900 to 1,000 individuals. Half of the visits are made in the home and half in the nursing clinic at the outpost. Medical consultation and/or referrals are sought on approximately a quarter of the patients seen. Experience has taught us that this is the maximum load a nurse can carry adequately in terrain that is as rugged as is Leslie County.

The nurse at the outpost is prepared to diagnose and manage common health problems in the family, to provide prenatal, postpartal, and healthy-child care, including family planning, and if necessary to perform a home delivery. She combines treatment with prevention and health maintenance skills, and when indicated, refers the patient to the physician or other members of the health team. She has available to her medical directives which have been developed by the physicians with nursing collaboration. They have the joint approval of both nursing and medicine, and they provide guidelines regarding the action that a nurse may undertake in the management of specific conditions, including emergencies. They also specify the points at which she must consult with or refer to the physician.

The physician visits each outpost at least once a month to review and assist the nurse with problem cases and to see those patients who need medical care but find it difficult to come to the hospital. A Utilization Review Committee, consisting of one physician, two nurses, and a social service worker, visits each center every three months to review records and promote sound health care. A field nursing supervisor and a coordinating nurse help to keep the outposts' services coordinated with each other and with the hospital.

The hospital has an ambulatory care center, where a total of 23,000 patients are seen annually. It is operated on the same general principles as the nursing outposts, except that a physician is immediately available and it has more supportive and diagnostic facilities and services. Patients are screened by the nurse who does a preliminary diagnostic work-up to determine if the condition is one that she can manage with the use of the medical directives, or if medical consultation and/or referral is indicated. Approximately half of the general clinic patients are seen by the physician. In the midwifery clinics, which include prenatal, postpartal, and family planning services, approximately 12 per cent of the patients are seen by the physician in a given week. All midwifery patients have a routine medical work-up early in pregnancy and are seen by the physician again during the final month of pregnancy. This system permits the physician to devote more of his time to the care of those conditions which require his skill. He also becomes more involved in teaching consultation, administrative details, and community activities.

A total of 1,900 patients were admitted to the hospital during the last fiscal year for an average of 3.1 patient days. The hospital has a total of twenty-six beds and twelve bassinettes. Seven beds are reserved for midwifery and five for pediatrics. The hospital averages about 275-300 deliveries a year. Approximately 95 per cent of the deliveries are managed by the nurse-midwives. The nurse-midwife is qualified to assume complete responsibility for the care and management of uncomplicated maternity patients. Obstetrical consultation is sought when complications arise. The nurse-midwives may admit and discharge patients according to hospital bylaws and regulations. The family nurse may also admit patients for nursing observation and care for up to twelve hours according to medical directives. This lessens, very markedly, the demands made upon the physician.

Major illnesses like major surgery are referred to one of the regional hospitals or to the University of Kentucky Medical Center. In these situations, the hospital or out-patient department serves as a primary contact agent.

Mental health care is considered an integral part of the total services offered. Psychiatric patients are admitted along with the general medical patients and referred to the local community mental health center or to the state institution as indicated. Many of them returned home after three to five days of hospitalization, and state institutionalization is thus avoided. Follow-up care may be provided by one of the nurses from the Community Mental Health Center or by one of the district nurses. A regional psychiatrist is available to the county one day every two weeks. When care of the mentally ill was discussed and put up for vote at a local committee meeting, the members stated that mental health services had never been separated from general care and this should not be changed.

Much of the success of the Frontier Nursing Service is attributed to its life-long pattern of local citizen participation. Before Mrs. Mary Breckinridge started the service, she did an extensive survey of the area visiting the people in the homes to learn first-hand what the major problems were and what the people wanted. No outpost was built without local participation, and to this day, each outpost maintains an active local committee which participates in local planning and is consulted regarding any major changes in the total services offered. They are also actively involved in fund raising. Of the 154 people employed by the FNS, 112 are local citizens. This includes primarily hospital and clinic aides, clerical workers, and maintenance and housekeeping personnel.

Indigenous health worker programs such as are used in many of the OEO projects remain to be developed. In the past, the nurse taught a member of the family to take care of the sick in the home, and the grapevine system was very effective in home health teaching. Family ties are very cohesive and it is a rare occasion when a suitable member cannot be found either in the immediate or the extended family to assume this responsibility. However, the pattern is changing. Individuals are beginning to expect pay for taking care of a family member, and waning birth rates and an increase in outside jobs lessen the choices that are available; therefore, new patterns will need to be established.

Curently there is considerable controversy regarding the type of worker that would be best suited for the system that has been developed by the FNS. To introduce a family health worker into the system to assist the family nurse would seem premature at this time. Until the areas of responsibility for primary health care provided by the family nurse have been more clearly defined and legal sanction established, it would only add to the confusion. Consideration has been given to the training of a home aide, rather than a health worker. The difference is subtle but highly significant.

Nursing aides offer valuable services in both in-patient and out-patient areas at the hospital, but attempted use of their services has not been as successful in the districts.

The development of clerical assistants, who have been taught some of the technical procedures, has been more successful. Several high school students who have worked in these capacities have gone on for further education, some in nursing and some in secretarial work. Few of those, however, return to the area after they complete their training. The use of the indigenous workers is a possibility that needs further exploration.

Professional personnel are recruited primarily from the areas beyond the mountains. Most of them have a very special interest in the type of care provided by the FNS, and they come from all parts of the country. Many have had past experience in underdeveloped areas, and they bring with them a wealth of knowledge and experience. The FNS currently employs one physician who has her boards in family practice with vast experience in group practice; one physician who has his Doctorate in Public Health and has trained medical assistants in Ethiopia; and one physician with a Masters in Public Health training who has been very actively involved in family planning at the international level and has had considerable experience in program planning and development in rural areas. The nurses come from an equally varied background. All help to add new dimension to both the service and the training program.

The training program in family nursing which is offered at the FNS is an extension of the nurse-midwifery training program which was developed in 1939. A total of 360 nurse-midwives have graduated from this program. It is a program that has evolved out of need and experience and is service-learning oriented. It is designed to give students exposure to, as well as front-line experience with, the day-to-day problems of health care in rural areas. It also provides opportunities for testing what they are taught. The aim is to add breadth, depth, and relevance to their learning. Too many students in this day and age receive their training in a sterile classroom atmosphere, far removed from the problems which they need to understand first hand if they are to handle them effectively.

The program is divided into three trimesters. During the first trimester, they are taught diagnosis and management of common health problems, family health assessment, counseling, and utilization of community resources.

During the second trimester, they have basic midwifery, prenatal, postpartum, and child care, and family planning. During the third trimester, they have the option of taking advanced midwifery, which focuses on intrapartal care, obstetrical and gynecological problems, and management of the newborn, or they may select outpost nursing which focuses on community health, district management, and family dynamics and therapy. The physical, psychological, social, and cultural aspects of health and illness are given heavy emphasis throughout the program. Much of this is through tutorial instruction. Each trimester is fifteen weeks in length, and students have approximately ten hours of classroom instruction and thirty hours of clinical practice a week.

The program is exciting, and interests in this type of training are spreading rapidly. The FNS has a contract with Vanderbilt University School of Nursing for the development of a masters program in Family Nursing, and it is exploring University affiliation for baccalaureate credit for the certificate program which has been outlined above. The future looks bright for continued program development, but much work remains to be done if the family nurse is to play a significant role in improving the delivery of health services in rural Appalachia.

The problems presented at this conference are all too familiar to the Frontier Nursing Service. It has known each one of them intimately besides knowing more. Perhaps the most crucial one is the survival of the small community agency. It cannot afford to compete with the larger agencies for federal funding, and it is becoming increasingly difficult to operate without such support. On the other hand, the small agency is vital to the community for the provision of primary health care. It is essential to the mountaineer that health services be provided at a personalized level, in a manner and at costs which are comparable to other services in the area, the latter because of his own limited income, and the former because of his life style which places high value on human relationship and a lesser value on commodities. Local planning which takes these factors into consideration is, therefore, vitally important.

The degree to which local planning becomes a matter of meeting the requirement and recommendations of federal, state, and regional agencies and conforming to regional planning rather than to meeting local community needs is frightening. It is over six years since the FNS first began negotiating with the federal agency to build a new health facility. It is still waiting final approval of its plans. The amount of time, effort, and money that has been expended on the planning is astronomical in comparison to the cost of the facilities to be built. The aim was to help the FNS avoid unnecessary costly expenditures. The result is a considerably more expensive facility than originally planned. The propriety of such planning is highly questionable.

The problems that rise out of isolation and poverty are difficult to fathom for someone who has not had exposure to them, and even more difficult to resolve without first-hand experience with them. The solutions require a system with a high degree of ingenuity, adaptability, and flexibility that is based on a knowledge of the area, its people, and its resources. Yet the small health agency, often with years of successful experience, is constantly confronted with rules and regulations that were formulated by others who have had neither exposure to nor experience with the problems of isolation and poverty. The day-to-day health problems encountered by the small health agency cannot be successfully managed through remote control; they require greater local autonomy than the state, regional, and federal systems currently permit.

The services provided by the larger, highly organized agencies tend to alienate the mountaineer; he often remains a stranger to them, turning to them only when in dire need. Yet the small agency, which can more readily remain individualized in its care, faces a continual struggle in its attempt to maintain a service that is relevant to local needs and that at the same time continues to meet the demands of the official agencies. The small agency finds itself continuously suspect as it attempts to compromise between the two without making cost prohibitive. This is a demoralizing process that is difficult to combat.

Not only is there lack of consideration for local needs at the state and national levels, but opportunities for constructive initiative action at the local level are often stifled. Minimum standards have been established by the elite for the elite. They do not take into consideration the existing standards and value systems within individual communities. Nor is there sufficient appreciation of attempts at self help. The small agency is thus becoming increasingly inundated by the federal and state agencies. The small agencies cannot afford the expertise of the government; they cannot fight its centralization and concentration of power; nor can they penetrate its insulation. To ask for increased federal support may therefore lead to the demise or strangulation of the smaller agencies, leaving the mountain people strangers to even the simplest of health care services. To counteract this, a system needs to be developed that permits much greater self-determination at the local level.

Chapter 10

HUMAN NEEDS AND THE AMERICAN
WELFARE SYSTEM

LESLIE DUNBAR

A GENERALLY agreed upon fact about American life in the 1960's and now the 1970's is that our welfare system is a failure. Almost as widely agreed is that, with proper reform, the system can be made to work.

If there is unanimity as to the fact of failure, there is very widespread and even harsh disagreement as to the explanation of the failure. If there is agreement that the system could be made to work, the prescriptions vary from greater severity toward welfare recipients to unfettered and sizeable guaranteed income. I would not question at all the conclusion that the welfare system is and has been a failure. I think we do, however, need to raise a question, even in the face of that optimism which is still an American characteristic, as to whether the system can be made to work at all; or, to be more to the point, whether we can reasonably expect it will be made to work. I would raise that question in recognition of at least six facts about American life and politics today.

The first of those is that we simply do not know what the American situation would be without a munitions economy. Those economists who tell us that the system can function perfectly well and perhaps even better without a heavy outlay for military projects do not base their message on empirical data, because there is none. Except for a quite short period of demobilization after the Second World War, we have had no experience since 1939 or 1940 with an economy not heavily supported by enormous outlays for munitions. During two periods, the Korean and now

126

Vietnamese,* it has been an economy heavily undergirded by huge war-making expenditures.

The question that faces us is twofold. One part is, can the welfare system be made to work while this goes on? The second is, what will be the prospects for a welfare system if our present military policies are finally curtailed and abandoned?

I think the answer to the first question is a flat no. I think that the energy that we may put into seeking a better welfare system, concurrent with the maintenance of approximately as large a military expenditure as we have been used to for the last decade, is and will be self-defeating; although, in the interests of the poor themselves, efforts to reform should not be discouraged, but we should not expect any radical or even marked improvement. At best, we may hold our own on the treadmill. I think they are doomed to fall short (and therefore the problems are doomed to become worse) because it is impossible to conceive of this or any society supporting the poor, in the numbers with which we have to deal in the United States, at a level of decency and adequacy while at the same time billions are nonproductively devoured by munitions for ourselves, for our client states and other dependencies, for foreign adventures, and for war. It is not simply a matter, and never has been, of guns versus butter. That has always been a fallacious mode of statement. It has never been a question of whether a country can afford butter as well as guns. The question always is whether we will afford both, and we will not. Even beyond is the fact that, although butter may be relatively a constant, guns are not. Guns always breed the need for more guns. So it is a question of whether you can have butter at the same time as you are having a constantly accelerating requirement for guns, and I think that the answer is clearly no.

So it would be wrong for us to encourage the belief that we can continue as an imperial power on a global scale, and, at the same time, make decent provisions for our poor, because we are not about to do that.

---

*The first adjective is probably inapt, but the second is not. As surely as other periods can be called, e.g. the Progressive period or the New Deal period, so the years since 1965 are the Vietnamese period of the Republic's history.

The second part of the question is whether, in the absence of
or having once overcome the policies that dictate militarism, we
can turn ourselves into the sort of economy that will have room
in it for the poor and will have within it the capability of elevating
the poor out of their present status. That, I think, is an unanswer-
able question at the present time given the present status of our
empirical knowledge of the American economy and the forces
operating within it.

Can the American economy (which we popularly though
rather vaguely call "capitalist" and "free enterprise") generate
adequate economic opportunities for some 20 or 25 million
people, having in the past failed to do so? Some of the commenta-
tors reinforce the widespread Puritan (or capitalist) ethic on this
point and blame poverty on the poor. William Ryan, in his new
and very good book of the same title, has named this "blaming
the victim." Unless we want to persist in triumphant Puritanism
and blame the victim, we have to see our millions of poor as the
product of our much vaunted economy.* If Keynesians can claim
to have solved the business cycle, they cannot, at least in America,
even claim to have proposed a plausible solution to the problem
of persistent poverty for those many millions of our countrymen
to whom poverty has never been cyclical, but a permanent historical and present fact.

Now it is unfortunately necessary to point out that the orgy
of governmental consumption that we have experienced since the
end of the Second World War and particularly in recent admini-
strations, has depleted our natural resources in a way that can only
render it less probable that this economy can generate a decent,
adequate life for all of its inhabitants.

If this is to be accomplished, it will require a newfound political maturity on the part of our people and political leadership of
a very high order, both by persons outside government and by
those granted political power. The same condition applies to the
ensuing questions of this chapter: without civic maturity and
leadership we shall have a desperate time meeting them.

---

*I say "triumphant," because in the seventeenth century there was another form
of Puritanism, represented in England by such as the Levellers, Diggers, and early
Quakers, who never subscribed to any such ethic.

I quickly add that when I speak of political "leadership," I do not tack on the fashionable adjective "charismatic." I have seen in my half-century enough too much, political charisma; I want no more. We can want dignity, courage, courtesy, compassion, stamina, clarity of purpose, openness of mind, a habit of respecting facts, an habitual respect for freedom and law.* We can want and need all these but we do not need the mystique of a charisma; we do not need leaders who themselves become causes, and thereby add to the problems and not to the solutions.

Second, we need to ask whether or not any reforms can be made to work, in light of the American practice of well-nigh total irresponsibility for the introduction of new technologies; for indeed, the high incidence of governmental subsidies of innovations, which, once brought to fruition, are allowed to pass without additional controls into the economy, regardless of their impact on human lives or the human capability of making a living. The facile proposition on which most of us have been reared, that there is no such thing as technological unemployment, or at worst it is only a transient thing, has to be questioned, not only regarding what is traditionally and precisely called technology but regarding the whole array of chemical, electronic, and other man-made inputs into the way we produce products and provide services. While it may be true that new technologies breed a satisfactory supply of jobs, the jobs too often are not for the people displaced. The problem of American poverty is precisely a problem of distinct groupings of people side-tracked by an ever-expanding economy and seemingly insulated from its opportunities.

Third, in the United States we are attmepting to do something (unconsciously, as usual) which so far as I know has never been done, not at least in Western history, unless possibly in the declining days of Rome. We are attempting to contain all of our poor within cities. The British enclosure movement and our southern plantations, while in both cases rendering the poor powerless, deprived, and even depraved, nevertheless allowed a great many of them to stay on the land and take their sustenance from it. The American system, since the farm policies of the New Deal and,

---

*As an example Clement Attlee could be described as the preeminent Western statesman of the twentieth century.

then, greatly accelerated by the technological revolution on the
farm in the 1950's and 1960's, has not only repeated and maintained the evils of enclosure and the plantation, but has literally
rendered the land uninhabitable for millions and millions of the
poor. There is no very clear prospect of that trend being curtailed,
though one of the truly good developments of our time is the
growing struggle of black Southerners to stay on the land. The
problems of the poor become, unless we decisively reverse the
trend, synonomous with the problems of the cities.

Fourth, one may hope this can be seen as something that will
as yet pass, nevertheless it is still true, as it has been for decades
of American history, that the Congressional committees, which is
to say the Congressional power, that deal with and apply themselves to the needs of the poor, are dominated by persons who
have not only a lack of concern and sympathy for the poor but
who manifest antagonism: the Senate Finance Committee, the
House Ways and Means Committee, the House and Senate Agricultural Committees, and the Agriculture Subcommittee of House
Appropriations. These, far more than the relatively liberal welfare and labor committees of the two houses, determine the shape
of legislation, appropriations, and even administration. In each
of those five committees there are attitudes and thoughts triumphant that could be fairly attributable only to a kind of know-noth-
ingism which the persons of Poage, Russell Long, Ellender, and
Whitten demonstrate continuously that we have not, as a people,
outgrown.

A fifth fact, that chills any optimism over the feasibility of reform, may also be a passing phenomenon. I would submit that it
is nevertheless true that, as of the present and as lasting beyond a
point that we can now see, the welfare crisis* in the United States
coincides with the collapse of our capability to manage large systems. The same country which cannot manage a welfare system,

---

*I believe this is correct usage. A crisis has been reached: there will be some marked
change. Liberals are not the only physicians on hand, however. The systematic
reform of our welfare system may be by the Reagans, Russell Longs, and Republi-
cans of the New York legislature. If so, it does not follow that their reforms will
not work, in the sense of lasting for a number of years; the discontents of the
poor can be, if a government wishes, fairly easily contained.

cannot manage its post office; the same country which cannot manage a commuter railroad system, cannot manage its metropolitan hospitals. We are not a very efficient country any longer. That thing which we most prided ourselves on possessing, viz. "know-how," turns out to be something we haven't much of anymore. Until we can recapture the capability of managing large systems efficiently, I see no reason to assume that we can reform that one system, the welfare system, for which there is the least interest on the part of the beneficiaries of American society.

Sixth, the poor are, nevertheless, caught in a vortex of enormous systems of power, wherever they turn. They deal mainly with huge institutions, which however badly or well managed are strong and overpowering in relation to them. Their lives are worked out, lived, and spent in a contest with huge hospitals, huge school systems and their huge bureaucracies, huge unions, huge welfare systems, huge housing authorities, and so forth; and increasingly, with huge commercial enterprises such as the supermarkets and the insurance companies and the agri-business employers. Hardly do any of these structures have within them career ladders which reward those who serve the poor effectively.

The above observations are not intended to overwhelm the question. They are not intended to put the question into a frame of reference which overlays it with insuperable problems. They are, however, intended to induce some realism, to say that maybe the questions are bigger than we would like to believe, and to say that we do need to raise radical issues if we in any sufficient measure will meet the challenge of these times. It should be clear to all of us as, I think, one of the key historical facts of the present day, that we are no longer doing what the sociologists used to speak of as "creaming." We are dealing with those persons who are actually at the bottom of the economic and social heap. That is what was always implied in the call of the early 1960's for integration, although seldom was it recognized. We were talking about something which was virtually impossible within the terms that liberals liked to believe. The old southern populists talked of putting the bottom rail on top; in our time the bottom rail is truly the bottom rail. It is that which all society rests upon, a kind of sub-foundation for the American social, economic, and political structure. It is simply impossible to integrate a foundation stone into the rest of a structure without shaking up the structure. That is to say, it is impossible to talk intelligently about integration without talking about radical issues, changes at the roots of the American life.

The above considerations also point to the conclusion that the welfare system cannot be successfully reformed in isolation from other determinants of the situation of the poor. Again, they point to the inescapable need for maturity and leadership. Without those qualities, we are sure to lose, and this national civilization should be seen now as on its decline. With those qualities, we have a chance.

I think it is likely that a society such as the United States will not undertake a long, deep-reaching reform of its welfare system more often than once in a generation. If that is the likelihood, then it behooves us to do it well. If the present is the time when forces are in confluence toward reform, it would be wise for us not to accept measures which may seem propitious to the politics of a particular year, because what we accept may very well be what we have to endure for another long stretch.

Although the weightiest opinion on this point should be that of the National Welfare Rights Organization, I would suggest that the two requirements of a minimally acceptable reform are as follows: a) the complete federalizing of costs, benefits, and criteria; and b) the guarantee that under any state plan no individual would receive less than is now being received from all sources.

The Welfare System must be federalized, root and branch, though not necessarily in the administration of it if that administration is carried on under explicit and sufficient federal criteria. I would carry the federalizing of financing and benefits to the point of flatly prohibiting any kind of state or local financial contribution supplementing the federal figure. I would have just one, single federal scale of payments with no regional differentiation.

Such a scale, of course, would have to be based upon need in the area where needs are most costly. That would, of course, mean that welfare recipients living in the South and some other districts of the country would have an advantage. I would let them have that advantage. There is no completely satisfactory way of spelling out regional differentials. More importantly, there is at the present time a real case to be made for an incentive for the poor to remain in and return to low cost areas.

Several years of talking with welfare recipients have made clear to me that, from their point of view, one of the primary wrongs is the nature and style of administration. The administration of welfare becomes an adversary relationship. Federalizing the finances, benefits, and criteria will go a great way toward altering that. Probably even more would be added by bringing recipients themselves into responsibility for much, if not all, of the local administration.

It is and has been my own conviction that the best form of welfare administration would be through a negative income tax. If we adopted that course, administration would become a routinized affair handled by the Internal Revenue Service (which would finally give a modicum of justification to keeping welfare in the jurisdiction of the House Ways and Means and the Senate Finance committees). There still would be a need for services of a social work nature, and the recipients themselves, with training as needed, would seem the best possible persons to give these.

The welfare payment, whether by negative income tax or other forms, should replace food stamps with cash. Perhaps some future generation will see food as a commodity which men should have solely because of need without the necessity to bargain and contend for. On that day, a universal voucher procedure might enhance efficient distribution. However, as long as ours is a cash economy, food stamps (or, for that matter, proposed new forms of vouchers such as rent certificates) are inappropriate.

Employment of welfare recipients (or the employment of persons who would be on welfare if not so employed) to provide most of the needed social work services would be consistent with what seems to me (and to many others, though, sadly, not to all) one of the few hope-inspiring contemporary developments, viz.

the movement sometimes though inaccurately called community control, sometimes though too grandly called participatory democracy. The movement has reached to health services, schools, and now in some places to law enforcement. It would seem to me an easy, and characteristically American, proposition that people should be encouraged and, most certainly, allowed to assume responsibility for the large institutions that often dominate their lives.

It is obvious that welfare is only one aspect of the life of the poor, interconnected with many others. Certainly it must be made coherent with the government's policies and programs in public health, education, housing, Social Security, minimum wage, and all the other governmental programs, whether federal, state, or local, which have central applicability to the poor.

Health and education are far more difficult to provide and administer than welfare, which requires nothing more than a cash payment. Health and education, on the other hand, require many highly trained professionals and other workers, vast facilities, and continuous personal contact. Traditionally, our schools have been available to all at little or no cost, and our health services have been similarly available to only what we call "charity patients." Despite this difference, the poor today seem about equally estranged from and ineffectively served by both systems. This suggests that the problems go deeper than the mode of financing. I certainly have not the omniscience to say anything very useful about those problems. Without much wisdom at all, however, one can say that the situation must surely require over the next few years the discovery of respect for each other and of ways of working together in some equality—by both professionals and clients.

The Citizens Board of Inquiry into Health Services for Americans concluded:

> The power of the consumer to control and influence the delivery system must be exercised at every level of the health care system: facility, service system or program, and neighborhood, city, state, region or nation. This power should include, but not be limited to, making policy, controlling assets (including expenditures), facilities, equipment and services. This does not mean that consumers will usurp the doctor's responsibility for meeting his patient's medical needs. On all

levels of decision-making, clear lines between policy (the consumer's primary business) and professional judgment regarding the individual patient (the physician's primary business) should be established.

In the final analysis, the people must remember, or learn, how absolutely necessary and yet how fragile is that layer of knowledge which protects and civilizes us. And, professionals need to remember, or learn, that professionalism has to be earned, that it derives from people's confidence, that it cannot be exacted by force, bluster, high prices, or the withholding of service.

We need to understand that when we talk about the welfare system, we are talking about human beings and their lives, we are talking about children and their chances to grow and to find some joy in life and to find some ways to fulfill themselves. We need to know that unless the system is humane and permeated by a concern for humanity, its efficiency is hardly of importance. Therefore, we need to know, among other things, that it is going to be expensive to provide a humane, decent welfare system for the poor of this country, who are poor in numbers that are not of their own making, but the making of this system. Before any kind of approach is made to reform our welfare system, there needs to be an understanding of how our economy failed so badly to have created this immense problem. I think that in asking that question we shall inevitably come, as part of the answer, to the fact that the American economic, political, and social system has never, historically, thought of the poor as deserving of respect: self-gratifying charity, perhaps, but not respect, and, in particular, not the poor who are black and brown. It will be costly, though in the long run (and not very long at that, probably) less costly than our present system. Among other things, this suggests that we must closely examine the tax structure to make sure that it is genuinely progressive, and that those revenues to which the public should legitimately be entitled are being collected.

The thrust of the Family Assistance Plan and the thrust of the proposals of the National Welfare Rights Organization, as well, have been toward income maintenance and away from job creation. When I say, as I do now, that I think job creation should be a principal thrust of our welfare program, I do not at all slight the need for income maintenance, as required and whenever needed. The handicapped, whether by age, illness, blindness, or whatever, should not be an issue for discussion. Rather, their needs should be met graciously and sufficiently by the public.

Nor would I, in any way, destroy or threaten the option of the mother who is a welfare recipient to decide what are the best interests of her children. That responsibility we must, far from destroying, seek to enhance. As the middle class mother decides what is in the best interests of her children and of herself, whether or not it is better for her to work in order to supplement the family income or to fulfill herself or to be better able to enrich the lives of her children, the mother on welfare should also have that responsibility and that option.

These are the kinds of recognitions that are dictated simply by need. I want to speak, however, to another kind of recognition which is not dictated by need, but by the hope for a better country, and by an estimation of what an individual wants and seeks in life. Unless my estimation is very, very wrong, there needs to be for most of us, (for, I would think, an overwhelming number of us), opportunities to feel useful and serviceable in this society in which we live.

A tragic truth about America's poor is that they are dispensable. If most of the welfare recipients, perhaps all of them, suddenly vanished overnight, society would be rid of an enormous burden, the productive work of society would go on about the same, and we would really quite likely be better off, given our present economic and social alignments. I think some realization of this must bear upon the poor, some crushing, heart-rending realization of their dispensability. If that is not calculated to infuriate a person and kill the spirits of a person, I do not know what is. If we are serious about opening up opportunities for humane living, then we must take seriously the needs of job creation. Moreover, if we truly desire to break the cycles of poverty and of urban ills which have plagued this country, then I think we must permit persons to choose whether they shall stay where they are or move. In either case there should be opportunities attracting and holding people to the city or to the rural area where they reside. It is not an answer to the problems of the poor to say, "Move; you no longer can make it where you are and we no longer can provide a way for you to make it where you are." I remember a federal official saying once to me that a person has no right to his residence. I think a person does have that right. As a matter of fact, it is even economic today for society to create jobs where the people are, rather than force them into a disruption of their lives and a consequent disordering of society by going elsewhere. I am not proposing that people be tied to any place. American society has always been a mobile society, and that opportunity for mobility should not be diminished. But, those who want to stay where they are should have the chance to do so.

Because we are so quick to misunderstand each other on these matters, I repeat that I am not talking about forcing or requiring mothers or, for that matter, able bodied men to work. I am speaking of the obligation of this society purposefully to create options. Nor am I talking about the creation of millions of broompushing, bedpan emptying jobs, nor of the subsidy of middle class home and marginal industries by supplementing the wages paid domestics and menials. What I am proposing is the creation of jobs (whether by the Department of Labor or HEW seems immaterial) that hardly anyone today is performing, such as a variety of services for preschool children; the management of neighborhoods in such matters as sanitation, recreation and public safety; nutrition counseling; the restoration of the environment; the cultivation of folk arts, perhaps in conjunction with the public libraries; lay advocacy and the manning of information offices; and many more that a resourceful public which does nothing more than consult its own needs will readily invent.

If we are going to take job creation seriously, we are going to have to think in terms of not just establishing industries here and there, but of creating a whole new variety of careers. To provide those jobs where people live, then we must have job policies that are flexible and administered by persons who have an intimacy with those parts of the country and with the lives of the people there.

For the past four decades, the small family farm has been

assaulted by economic, technological, and even governmental forces. One does not have to be a sentimentalist to note that the poor are today largely cut off from the chance of making a living from the land. There is plenty of that: the countryside begins to look deserted. Resettlement is probably not feasible or even desirable. Governmental policies and subsidies that make it possible for a family to be self-reliant on a farm are both feasible and desirable.

Our farm policies are contrary to the interests of the poor. Our farm policies have been one of the notable failures of American history. By any criterion, the policies established by Congress and Presidents in the twentieth Century have been monumental failures. If one applies to them any of the obvious tests, the answer is that they have failed. They have not defended the family farm, indeed, they have been a powerful inducement to the collapse of the family farm. They have not enabled people living on the land to make a living, indeed, they have helped to drive millions and millions of people off the land. They have not protected the interests of farm labor, indeed, they have always been chary of recognizing that farm employees had any interests that the law should acknowledge and protect. They have begrudgingly and occasionally adopted conservation as an interest, but never one that equals the interest of profit-taking when the two come into conflict. They have not been in the interest of the consumer, because they have been an encouragement to lower and lower nutritional and taste standards in the food we grow and sell to ourselves. Farm policies in the United States have come to have as their overriding purpose the maximization of the income of the producers of basic crops. Insofar as that has been the purpose, and it is, those policies have been contrary to the interests of the poor. We need to restudy very seriously the agricultural policies and powers, the agricultural committees of Congress, and the Department of Agriculture. They must end their warfare against the poor and their slavish services to the giants of agri-business.

No program of job creation or of community participation in the administration of services is likely to be at all successful, and indeed should not be accepted, unless it is consistent with the gains that organized labor has established for itself, in regard to wages, hours, and conditions of work. This does not necessarily mean that we must turn to organized labor to write the programs. It does mean that those who do write them should do so with a protective eye on the gains made by the poor of a previous generation. On the other hand, where organized labor stands athwart the path that those who are still poor must take for self-development, it blocks their portals. Those liberals who excuse the unions for doing so are among the *de facto* conservatives and obstructionists of our time.

It is commonplace to point out that the American poor of the 1970's consists, in its largest proportion, of persons who were the victims of systematic oppression by institutions of American life during the history of the Republic. That was true of the blacks, all of whom are the descendants of slavery. It is also true of the Appalachian whites, who have been victimized by this country's demand for coal and by the rapacious, lustful, inexcusable methods by which we mine it. It is true of the Mexican-Americans of the Southwest, who have been in many instances defrauded of their land and made inferior subjects by conquerors. It is true of the American Indians. History can hardly be repealed. What the poor can ask is that the oppression stop, but it has not stopped. The poor need not only the services of government; the poor need the cessation of those policies and acts of government and other "power" institutions which continue deliberate oppression and exploitation. The poor of Appalachia need to have the strip mining, which renders their land uninhabitable, stopped. The poor of developing urban centers in the South need to have government stop building expressways that destroy their neighborhoods. The poor of Harlem need to have government stop building incinerators and dumps virtually in their backyards. The poor of Texas and the American Southwest generally need to have government enforce its own laws and close the border, because as long as the border is open there is little chance of farm workers holding their own. Those same farm workers need to have government stop cooperating with their opponents in labor disputes by such practices as great purchases of grapes by the Department of Defense. The poor in every part of the country need to have governments stop violating their civil liberties.

Why do we go on talking about how to deliver health services to the poor? The very word "deliver" tells the sad tale. People, in the nature of things, either have to come to health services or have the services brought to them. Either way, money and some power are required. In Appalachia, the poor are kept poor and relatively powerless. They will, therefore, stay unhealthy; poor people always do. They are kept poor by coal and oil companies and all others which mine and misuse the wealth and spirits of the mountains. The answers to the health problems of Appalachia lie in the legislatures and courts of West Virginia, Kentucky, Tennessee, Virginia, and, above all, the United States. As long as those legislatures and courts permit the devastation of the region's natural and human resources, ill health and physical misery and even mental underdevelopment will characterize the poor of this region.

The recent White House Conference on Children provided only the latest documentation of the torment which is life in America for the children of the poor. The Comprehensive Child Development Bill (H.R. 6748, S. 1512) would go a long way toward changing that. In addition to that, the states and municipalities, which are responsible for the schools, the juvenile courts, the training schools, the whole apparatus of institutional suffocation, have a lot to answer for.

Again, we should acknowledge that there are literally no solutions to American poverty that do not include jobs. To place priority on child welfare appeals to our hearts, and also to our felt need for a beginning point at which to break the cycle of poverty. I think it will not do, not, at any rate, unless we desire taking a sizeable step in the direction of totalitarianism. If not, we shall continue to rely on families for the rearing of children. The family is held together by a vocation or vocations. Seen in this aspect (and many of the poor do so see it) the current emphasis on children's rights and child welfare can appear as one more sellout, one more double dealing, or at best, one more grotesque irrelevancy, unless accompanied by an equal and prior emphasis on jobs and income.

Last year, there was a great deal of talk about breakthroughs, about new principles. The American tradition has been, as I suggested above, always one of scant support, and throughout our history a tradition of saying that the poor must get by on something less than all the rest of us acknowledge as being the minimum required for a decent existence. Coupled with our charity has been our rebuke, and our way of rebuke has been to give short supply. We must not overclaim for any reform proposals that are made; therefore, we must not indicate conviction that a new system once started will improve each year. That is not certain to be the case. Unless we now completely federalize the system, it is not even likely to be the case. Once in a generation do we have a probable chance to reform welfare. There will be no new principle in the American welfare system that does not break the old tradition.

There will be no new principle unless we adopt a principle of adequacy, a principle that the poor are human beings who, therefore, need to be treated with respect, which is to say they need to be afforded the chance of dignity from their childhood on.

Some years ago, the social psychologists taught that behavior and attitudes were separable, and that in such matters as race it was not necessary to change people's attitudes; it was necessary to change only their behavior. We learned well from the social psychologists, and much of the thrust of the reform movement of the 1960's was away from the older notion that peoples' hearts and minds had to change, and was directed along the lines of this new strategy to bypass, as it were, hearts and minds and concentrate instead on the way people acted. There was much to be said for that strategy, and it accomplished a great deal. Like all strategies, it has its limitations, and I suspect some years ago we reached the limitations of this one, though we have been slow to recognize that we did.

It is true today, as it has been for the past five or six years, that many of the legistative and other institutional advances made in civil rights and race relations are not accepted thoroughly in the minds of multitudes of people, and it is, to a very large extent, those minds and the attitudes which they generate which will have, as they are having, the primary impact on the kind of nation we are and will become. The Congress of the United States, the Presidents of the United States, the civil rights leaders, and other such persons have less to say, I think, about the kind of nation we shall become than do millions of voters, millions of parents of school children, millions of home owners, millions of churchgoers, and so forth, making up their minds, making their own individual policies as to where they shall live, with whom they shall go to church, and where they shall send their children to school. This is all to say that there is a task of a magnitude which can very well overwhelm us, or at least discourage our efforts. It may, nevertheless, be the demand of realism that we turn again to find ways of educating the American people. In no field is that more necessary than in welfare. We must acknowledge the fact that probably most persons not on welfare do not sympathize with the needs of those persons who are on welfare; that most persons not on welfare are all too prone to believe the worst about those who are; and that most persons not on welfare are unhappy with the use of their taxes to support other people. Those persons not on welfare are likely, for any number of reasons, to feel vengeful or punitive or merely censorious of those persons who are. This is a tremendous challenge to national leadership. It is too much to ask the National Welfare Rights Organization or the Southern Christian Leadership Conference to carry the burden of interpreting the problems of welfare to the middle class of the United States. The rest of us are in a better position to do so, and have far greater responsibility.

On the other hand, there is the question of the content of such public education, and here we must reflect that a nation seldom learns what its history and culture do not prepare it to learn. Fortunately, American culture does have a predisposition toward what could be the essential lessons anyway. We are habituated to legalism and to the enshrinement of abstract principles. We may very well be beating dead horses when we seek to redirect national priorities on the basis of appeals to save "the city," in whose survival and prosperity too few of the influential middle class acknowledge an interest, and which the white working class apprehends to be passing with the political control of blacks.

A far more radical (*i.e.* basic) , and paradoxically, quite possibly more popular, appeal would call for a definition and assertion of minimum national standards of education, health, nutrition, housing, etc., below which no individual child or adult would be allowed to fall; and a concomitant translation of such standards into legal rights that a person could speedily invoke in courts in his or her own behalf. "Standards" is the sort of abstract concept that American minds are used to accepting; legally defensible individual rights are at the very core of our political methodology.

If we federalize welfare, in particular if we give it the neutral appearance that it would have as a negative income tax, we would remove some and probably much of the provocative aspect of the deteriorating relations between the welfare recipients and the lower wage and salary earners. These latter people, who are constantly and necessitiously preoccupied with the cost and the adequacy of health, housing, schools, etc., would benefit as well as the poor from the establishment of standards.

Standards will be of slight help, however, if they cannot be legally required and enforced. To do this there must be a) a great expansion of the number of lawyers publicly supported and in the public service; or b) the invention of new offices such as lay advocates, and new tribunals and processes for settling claims; or c) both more lawyers and new methods. Such lawyers and advocates, if they are to serve well the purpose of enforcing standards in the interest of the individual, will have to be client-controlled, which is, unfortunately, not the direction many of our new breed of public interest lawyers are traveling.

We must not, however, expect more from dispute settling tribunals than they are likely to give. It is precisely in those areas, where the many are dispossessed of all power and the few monopolize it, that the courts are frequently at the service of money and power: neither they, nor new tribunals, will consistently or even often "tell truth to power." We need, therefore, to have an openness to, a readiness to accept, emerging forms of community organizations. OEO's greatest contribution has been its encouragement of this. We should not try to predict or direct the form community organizations or community unions will take.

We should look upon their growth as a movement basically good and necessary for establishing equitable relationships of power in our society.

I cannot conceive that, if we were talking about the reform of the labor laws of this country, we would not turn to the AFL-CIO, the United Auto Workers, or the Teamsters for advice and even leadership. I cannot conceive, if we were talking about the reform of farm policies of this country, we would not turn to the Farm Bureau and the Grange for advice and leadership. We do, however, when talking about the reform of our policy seldom turn to the poor themselves for advice, and never for leadership. I think we must begin to do that. In recognition of the centrality of the poor in today's health and educational picture, we must begin to do it in those areas as well.

It is not possible, of course, to do so except through organizations which have some validity in their claim that they represent the poor. The great achievement of the anti-poverty program was that it did, for a brief span of years anyway, provide the poor all over this country with a chance to build institutions that gave them some power over their lives, that gave them some chance to grow and develop as leaders.* In many Head Start centers, in many Community Action Agencies, and in co-ops, we have accumulated a reservoir of new leaders close to the poor because they themselves are of it, and a reservoir of fragile but still useful institutions. We have, besides, national organizations such as the National Welfare Rights Organization, the Southern Christian Leadership Conference, the United Farm Workers, Aspira of America, the National Congress of American Indians, and many local organizations of the poor. Great numbers of new leaders have appeared in these last ten or fifteen years, and to them we ought to turn for guidance and insight as to what are the requisites for successful as well as humane programs to fulfill human needs. There ought, at national, state, and local levels, to be councils of them as advisors and planners, helping design the

---

*Not to be overlooked is the fact that when the anti-poverty program worked well it accomplished that, but when it worked poorly, it created new power struggles and new competitions which have racked poverty communities.

shape of new systems, systems which would take as their purpose the treatment of every being as a person of humanity and dignity, entitled to respect and cooperation from each of us.

Chapter 11

WHAT IT WOULD TAKE FOR ME TO PRACTICE IN AN ISOLATED RURAL COUNTY

WILLIAM TAYLOR FITHIAN III

I FIRST WANT TO REGISTER my disappointment because there are very few physicians and instructors from the West Virginia University Medical Center attending this conference. Consider that only ten miles away there are about three hundred doctors who every day instruct us in what medicine is and what we should want to do with medicine; yet, when they do not seem to be interested in a thing like this conference, one really begins to question what it is all about.

I am feeling a great deal of anxiety at this moment for several reasons. First, because I believe I am one of those people Dr. Looff referred to as having a difficult time with verbalization. I have always felt a great deal more at ease being silent than I have when speaking, especially in front of such an audience as is here today.

Second, my anxiety level is at an all time high because I have not completely recovered from several of the comments made in earlier papers. I am referring particularly to the comment Dr. Miernyk made in regard to me. He said he was looking forward to my presentation on what it would take to get me to practice in an isolated rural county. He then said, whatever it would take, isn't there. Dr. Miernyk, the moment you said that I felt as though you had personally kicked me in the stomach. I am still gasping for air, but I have taken in enough to become angry at you and people like you.

Third, perhaps my greatest anxiety is my concern about my ability to effectively relate to you my sincerity. What I am ex-

146

pressing is very important to me. I do not want its importance diminished because of my inability to verbalize. One of my closest friends once told me that I have what he would call a tragic flaw in my personality—that tragic flaw is my inability to be much more than an idealist and my inability to believe in something without becoming emotionally involved. I hope today that my idealism and my emotionalism do not stand in the way of what I am presenting.

When Dr. Schwartz asked me if I would like to speak today on what it would take for me to practice medicine in an isolated rural area, I thought it would be rather simple to do, because practicing in a rural area was my goal during my premedical studies and my first couple of years in medical school. However, during the past few weeks, while reassessing my attitudes toward working and living in a remote rural area, I realized that many of my feelings and concepts about rural medicine had changed, and many of my ideas that had not changed were complex and involved. It has also been within these past few weeks that for the first time people have begun to ask me with any seriousness, "Do you really want to practice medicine in a rural area?" Consequently, this is also the first time I have had to defend my reasons and ideas with any conviction. It has been a combination of these events that makes me wonder now if I do want to practice and live in a rural area and, perhaps even more confusing and bewildering to me, if I am prepared to do so.

Maybe I can explain the dilemma in which I find myself by exploring some of the problems, ideas, and feelings I share with other medical students concerning medical education and health care, and, particularly, delivery of care.

In the May, 1971 issue of *Time* magazine, Dr. Tormey of the University of Vermont School of Medicine said, "the contrast between the senior class and the far more liberal freshman class is almost a generation gap within the student society itself. Many of the new students are interested in going to public health rather than a lucrative private practice." I believe this, to a large extent, describes our medical school here. There are vast differences among the students as a whole in the first couple of years from

those in my class. The differences, however, deal not so much
with an appearance that the seniors want a lucrative private practice and the freshmen and sophomores do not, but with the attitudes, motivations, and goals concerning how and where they
want to practice medicine and deliver health care.

A classmate of mine said he would be skeptical of any physician who at some time had not considered being a country doctor.
Yet he, as well as many others of my classmates, has drifted away
from that goal and they are looking forward to specializing and
practicing in sizeable metropolitan areas. Why has this happened?
It has happened partly, as I see it, because we have been led to
think that it is the highly specialized areas of medicine that we
should want to go into and it is this type of medicine we have
been taught. Except for some experience in Mexico, I have had
no exposure to health care in rural areas; few of my classmates
have either. For the most part my medical education has existed
within a very sophisticated, complex structure far removed from
the routine unsophisticated practice of medicine in a rural area. I
am sure the majority of my classmates know little about what it
would really be like as the country doctor most of us have
imagined at some time in our brief careers. This by itself limits us
in making a decision to practice medicine in a rural setting.

Then, too, I, like my peers, have drifted away from a rural way
of life. Although some of us were raised in small towns, during
our years of premedical training and medical school, we have
grown accustomed to living in larger cities. This, too, makes it
even more difficult to know if we are capable of returning to and
enjoying life in a rural area.

Again, in contrast, the majority of students in the first two
years seem to expect, demand, and require different things from
their medical education than I did. An example of this is a group
of first and second year students at West Virginia University who
are trying to initiate a free clinic in Osage, a small community
outside of Morgantown, which lacks health facilities.* These students have opened an avenue in which they hope to be able to ex-

---

*The Osage Free Clinic was established in April 1972.

plore the practice of medicine away from the setting of the Medical Center.

In addition to wanting more opportunities to learn about rural health care and delivery, the first and second year students differ to a large extent from my classmates concerning where they want to live. Several first year students, for example, have bought a fifty-acre farm in neighboring Preston County with the hope of returning there upon graduation to practice medicine.

Many of these newer students, as Dr. Tormey called them, are creating opportunities for themselves in medicine and are developing a life style while still in medical school that will make practicing in a rural area far more feasible upon graduation than it will be for myself or my classmates.

At this point you may feel uneasy: does he or doesn't he want to be a rural doctor? Indeed, it must be apparent that I am not sure. I am sure, however, that I am somewhere within what Dr. Tormey called "a generation gap within a student medical society itself." Even though I feel unprepared to make a knowledgeable decision about practicing in a rural community, I still want to work and live in a rural setting. Because of the type of medical education I have received and the pattern of life I have led, I feel I must place certain requirements on that rural area. These may be the same requirements that will affect those medical students now in the first couple of years of school, after further exposure to our medical education and to a life far removed from the rural setting.

The necessary conditions which I must consider in regard to any rural community in which I expect to practice involve essentially four fundamental areas:

1. Considerations of my family.
2. The community itself.
3. The professional community.
4. Access to a major medical center.

Family Considerations

Dean McKee recently stated at a class meeting that the most important factor in choosing our internships will be the attitude of our wives about the geographical location. I believe that he is right. I want my wife and eventually my children to be happy, content, and involved in any area in which we live. Dr. Spradlin, Chairman of the Department of Psychiatry at West Virginia University, said that the most essential element in one's medical career is the security of one's family. Since medicine is not going to be like a fraternity to me, the desires and needs of my family will be of utmost importance in determining where I practice medicine. My wife, for example, has a career of her own—one that is equally as important to her as medicine is to me. She has a right to pursue it. Consequently, any isolated rural area where I work must also provide her the opportunity to pursue her career. If the community itself cannot support my wife and her work, then there must be some adequate means by which she can commute to a larger city, whether this is through safe roads or commercial transportation.

When my wife and I think of an isolated community, we realize that it is not likely to have much in the way of libraries, theaters, or cultural activity. I believe that one can make up for these aspects of a rural area which are lacking if they are made accessible; again, this means having the free time and good roads to make it possible to travel to the larger cities.

Community Involvement

The second fundamental requirement entails many factors and involves the community itself. What type of rural community would appeal to me and my wife? It would have to be one whose members take an active part in the community itself. It would be a community that is willing to be an active participant in organizing and determining the type of health care it wants. I, as a physician, would not want to shoulder the entire burden of giving health care to a community. Such a community must want to initiate and improve its health facilities and participate in preventive medical programs. The community must, also, and this is very critical, be progressive in its attitudes toward schools and education. I cannot imagine living and raising my family in an area which regularly vetoes new funding for improving school facilities, acquiring teachers, increasing teachers' salaries, and strengthening the educational curriculum. The members of the community must also have, or at least develop, a strong social conscience towards the obligation they have to the natural environment. I do not want to live in any community that permits its rivers, recreational areas, and natural resources to be destroyed. Finally, the community must be willing to share in the responsibility to alleviate poverty in the area.

Professional Community

We then come to the third fundamental requirement relating to the professional community itself. Any isolated rural area is going to require more than a single physician to answer its health needs. It is going to need a health team and this encompasses not only the physician, but dentists, nurses, social workers, pharmacists, and other paramedical personnel. It would, I am sure, be useless for me to set up practice in a remote area if I did not have at my disposal these other resources to assist me in giving total patient care. It is total patient care that I am concerned with, not just treating acute ailments. If I were alone in a community, I would be professionally isolated, and in a short period I would be overworked, disillusioned, discouraged, and stagnated.

A professional community requires adequate hospitals and clinics. Each time I see a patient in need of hospitalization, I do not want to send him fifty to a hundred miles away. Part of the satisfaction of practicing medicine involves treatment and experiencing the recovery of the patient. This satisfaction would obviously be lost if facilities for the treatment of the patient were not a part of the rural community.

Medical Center Access

My final topic of discussion involves access to a major medical center. Isolation in a rural area would place numerous restrictions on me as a physician. I would not have immediate access to physicians who are specialists, to modern diagnostic and treatment techniques, or to the sources of information to which I have grown accustomed while in my medical training. I would miss and need many of these things. Unless it were possible for me to have access to them, I would again feel isolated and become apathetic. Here I do not simply mean access by good roads leading to the major medical center, but the feasibility of utilizing the medical center. There has to be a working relationship between a private physician in a remote rural area and the medical center itself. The major medical center must continue to be a source of support to the rural physician far more than to the physician who is practicing in a large metropolitan area where he is surrounded by many peers and facilities.

Things That Must Be Done

Now that I have expressed some of my feelings about practice in a rural area as well as some of my requirements, you may wonder whether I could practice medicine in an isolated area. Indeed, I have been negative in many areas and critical in others. However, considering what I indicated it would take for me to practice medicine in an isolated community, you will see that some of these requirements either can be met or already have been met. As far as my wife and her having an opportunity to pursue her career, she could if there were roads that would enable her to get to larger areas within a reasonable period of time. As to the community itself and its attitudes toward providing health facilities, good schools, and taking care of its natural environment, I am not sure. I do know that there are some communities in West Virginia, such as the town in the eastern panhandle of the state where I was raised, that are involved in developing their medical facilities, improving their schools, and seeking solutions to poverty.

With regard to the professional community itself, I am sure this could, in time, develop if the vicious circle of poverty, poor community involvement, lack of community facilities, and apathy were broken. Finally, the isolation of the rural physician need not be one of total isolation if means are made available to him to utilize and be an active member of a larger medical center. This is being done to a certain extent here at the University by the use of telelectures transmitted throughout the state and by periodic postgraduate refresher courses.

In summary much of the rhetoric used in describing what it will take for me to practice in an isolated rural area may have been redundant without facing the crises and issues that have been presented in other papers. I believe that I might have been better off by simply focusing on what it would take for me to practice in Appalachia, Dr. Miernyk, what it is that is there, is simply the need. It really is nothing more than my sense of responsibility and obligation which would make me practice in Appalachia.

But, in all honesty, I know that because of the way things are now in our rural communities, and because of the many changes our communities, our states, our medical schools, and our Federal Government must bring about, I cannot say at this moment that I will move to and begin work in an isolated area with any permanency in mind. I am planning, however, to be at least a transient physician in one of our rural areas—spending a few years there and then, if I and my family find it necessary, returning to one of the larger metropolitan areas. I am not sure how best I could be this transient physician. It may simply be as a private physician who periodically spends time in a rural setting, or as a member of the Public Health Service, possibly through the Emergency Health Personnel Act recently passed.

At this point I wish to quote from E. E. Cummings, with the hope that it will partly explain the situation in which many of us who are medical students find ourselves.

> To be nobody—but yourself—in a world which is doing its best night and day to make you everybody else—means to fight the hardest battle any human being can fight; and never stop fighting.

Chapter 12

FEDERAL ACTION NEEDED FOR RURAL HEALTH

ROBERT L. NOLAN

THE MANY problems in rural areas of Appalachia and other parts of the United States that are responsible for serious inadequacies in health care include the following: poverty—personal and institutional; isolation created by geography, weather and poor roads; population dispersion; weak public and private institutions; absence of transportation; unemployment; inadequate housing; discrimination; inadequate water supply; absence of waste disposal; severe shortages of health personnel; absence of health care facilities; poor educational systems; impassable roads; barriers to qualifying for existing benefits of public programs; inadequate welfare services; environmental pollution; adverse land use practices such as strip mining and uncontrolled timbering; attitudes of despair and depression; and maldistribution of health personnel.

Ultimately legislative action that is designed to permanently improve health and the quality of life in rural areas must be the product of a public policy committed to deal comprehensively with such issues.

Even in the absence of such a comprehensive attack, a variety of federal health legislation has been adopted or is now being considered that bears directly upon health care and services. In this brief review some of these federal legislative trends will be examined and some further proposals for legislative action and implementation made.

A recent Report of the United States Senate Government Operations Subcommittee revealed that federal health programs and spending is administered in twenty-four separate departments and agencies.

Most of these programs are not correlated or coordinated with each other. Officials in agencies with similar programs have been reported ignorant of other agency activity in the same field.

In the health manpower field, there are several dozen training programs administered by different agencies. These have given emphasis to increasing the quantity of health professionals by a combination of loans and grants to trainees, and grants for construction and expenses to educational institutions.

While such programs have undoubtedly increased both the availability of training in the health professions and the total supply of health personnel, there is still an acknowledged shortage of all professional categories in rural areas. None of these programs offers effective incentives to use these federally financed skills in health manpower shortage areas.

The President's recent proposal for loan forgiveness for new medical school graduates is an unlikely inducement for medical practice in rural areas when one considers the economic realities of opportunity elsewhere. Nor do new developments to federally finance training programs in family practice and new health professional categories offer any suggestion that graduates of these programs will apply their training in shortage areas.

Another major category of federal health programs involves direct health or related services ranging from relatively narrow categorical efforts providing for milk for school children to comprehensive health services development under section 314 (e) of the Public Health Service Act. Even within the framework of program priorities, allocation of benefits is largely dependent upon initiative and entrepreneurial efforts.

Another typical requirement involves matching funds from the local areas and sufficient personnel and existing services to offer a good prospect for success of the new program. Faced with shortages in regard to all these characteristics, the rural areas are less likely to see new direct health services made available to them despite their great needs.

The Appalachian Regional Development Act of 1965 is a unique effort to bring needed services of a high priority to this region. At least a dozen demonstration health programs including one in southern West Virginia are in operation now. However, despite the recognition of special Appalachian needs that generated this legislation, even here matching local funds are required for most of the categories in the Act. This continues to impede the areas in greatest need for qualifying for benefits or continuing their participation.

Health facilities construction programs administered by at least six different departments or agencies range from the familiar Hill-Burton efforts started in 1946 under the Public Health Service to the recent loan provisions administered by the Federal Housing Administration for development of group practice facilities. Matching funds are generally required for all of these construction efforts. While many of these facilities have been located in rural areas, the concentration of population and resources in urban areas also results in focusing these efforts in the cities and suburbs.

Construction of a facility, however, does not assure its availability to the poor in rural areas who lack necessary cash for hospital and medical care, nor necessarily attract personnel to staff the facilities. Empty, partially used, or economically inaccessible rural health facilities are scattered throughout the nation.

The Administration's anticipated proposal for satellite centers for teaching and health services in shortage areas could be a base for improving health delivery and relating programs to medical schools and regional centers near rural areas.

With the adoption of the Medicare and Medicaid programs in 1965, the Federal Government became the largest single source of payment for individual medical services. Earlier social security provisions had already provided for reimbursement to states for medical care costs for certain welfare recipients and categorically aided groups. Furthermore, as an employer the Federal Government in 1959 commenced contributions for prepaid health programs selected by their employees. All these efforts have had the common feature of providing payments for the existing system of health services. To the extent that these payment efforts have not been linked to system change, they have tended to reinforce the existing limitations. Although Medicare has provided the elderly in rural areas with a payment mechanism, it has not generated a network of available services near their homes. Medicaid programs which depend upon states to participate in financing have been unevenly and unequally applied, leaving many of the rural poor without any access to this payment device. The latest amendments initially approved in Committee would not disturb these basic payment characteristics, although other program changes including Medicare coverage of the disabled have been proposed.

The newest proposals for various health insurance approaches would extend a payment mechanism for health for most citizens. Some attention has been given in several of these proposals to inducements for program development or services in shortage areas. To what extent these could benefit rural areas is quite uncertain at this time. However, we have observed that both public and private financing mechanisms have thus far favored urban areas where there is a concentration of population, facilities, funds, and employment groups.

At the medical schools the availability in the past of funds for research rather than services has contributed to the proliferation of both a laboratory emphasis and specialization. The specialist model with the needed elaborate technical facilities and resources is the antithesis of the model needed to interest students in rural practice, as many schools now recognize. In addition the research emphasis in the past has not been directed toward the unique problems of rural health. For example, we still do not have an organized, continuing data collection system that identifies health characteristics in isolated rural areas.

Enactment of legislation by itself does not produce change. The implementation is the critical stage that requires a number of responsive characteristics in the organization. A number of developments in recent years have impaired the function of federal agencies that administer health programs. Among the problems manifest have been uncertainty about availability of funds, reorganization of roles and functions, changes in personnel, and sudden policy shifts. In some agencies it is not uncommon to return a call to an administrator who left the preceding week or find that a particular program has been suddenly curtailed, revised, or eliminated. In the politics of bureau priorities, rural health has suffered by absence of significant representation either in the agency organizational structure or on the boards and councils that determine who receives the funds.

In addition, most of these policies are determined in the setting of a large caged maze in Rockville (called the Parklawn Building) containing several thousand employees, almost as effectively hemmed in and remote from the problems of rural health as if they were prisoners at San Quentin. Concentration and isolation of the bureaucrats there may help process forms, but it does not offer a window to witness the health problems of people in rural areas.

Nevertheless, we must recognize that federal economic involvement is essential. As a noneconomist, absent some economic miracles, I personally can see no substantial improvement in health conditions in isolated rural areas without massive federal assistance.

In our experience in this region, many residents of isolated rural areas have considerable difficulty in qualifying for those federal programs and benefits that they are eligible for. The remoteness from health and social service agencies and the lack of local information and experience further deprives the rural individual of needed services.

When a categorical program such as family planning is available, it is difficult for the isolated lady in the "hollow" to understand that the program may be concerned with contraception, e.g. but cannot pay to keep her alive by excising her cervical cancer, so that she can survive to enjoy the benefits of planning her family.

It may be of special interest to note that President Nixon called attention to ". . . archaic laws in twenty-two states," which prohibit or limit group practice or limit the delegation of certain medical tasks. He has asked the Secretary of HEW to draw up a model statute to correct these anomalies, and has indicated that he will supercede them with contracts with Health Maintenance

Organizations which could then preempt any inconsistent state statutes.

RECOMMENDATIONS FOR LEGISLATIVE AND POLICY ACTION

The specific rural health problems that we have been discussing are subject to alleviation, if we really do intend to translate the current rhetoric into meaningful action. Among those legislative and policy steps which could make such a contribution, I would like to offer the following recommendations:

1. *Establishment of a major Rural Health Bureau within the Department of Health, Education, and Welfare,* with responsibility for developing, coordinating, and delivering programs in health and health related matters to people in rural areas.

2. *Adoption of a well-financed federal scholarship program in the health professions,* especially medicine, nursing, and dentistry, similar to new ones now offered by the armed services. This would provide not only full payment of tuition, books, and expenses, but the salary of or equivalent to a junior officer in the Public Health Service, which would range currently from 8,000 dollars per year (the first year) to 12,000 dollars per year, in the fourth year of training. In return for this scholarship the young medical graduates, for example, would have a five-year service commitment in health manpower shortage areas either as commissioned PHS officers in direct primary care in health manpower shortage areas or under other approved arrangements.

3. *Establishment of a National Clearinghouse for positions in health manpower shortage areas.* At present there is no central location for either communities in shortage areas or all the various individual health professionals to exchange information. It is proposed that there be established a national clearinghouse for positions in health manpower shortage areas within HEW. This clearinghouse would provide information and maintain listings of communities and areas with health professional needs as well as all prospective health workers interested. The service would be free and limited to health manpower shortage areas.

4. *Selective Service credit for rural health service.* Service in

health manpower shortage areas under prescribed conditions, whether as a uniformed officer of USPHS or under other conditions and regulations required by statute should provide full credit under the Selective Service Act and exemption from military service resulting from such service in health manpower shortage areas.

5. *Effective implementation of the Emergency Health Personnel Act of 1970 (PL 91-623).* The early innovative and imaginative implementation of this new law could enlarge the incentives for practice in health manpower shortage areas. Efforts to commence programs under this statute should be accelerated. Administrative units of the program should be located in rural and inner city areas, close to the problems and hopefully with more flexibility than usual. The emerging Appalachian Environmental Health Center in Morgantown is an example of an ideal rural location for the program in the Appalachian region.

6. *Provision of transportation arrangements for patients.* Legislation should be provided to assure adequate transportation for both diagnostic referrals, illness, and emergencies between homes, rural practitioners' locations, satellite clinics, regional medical centers, and medical school locations. Absence of transportation in rural areas cannot be remedied without direct federal support to eliminate this major obstacle to the provision and delivery of rural health services.

7. *Development of a referral network and communication techniques.* The Federal Government should devise appropriate mechanisms which will permit referral to medical centers such as medical schools, regional hospital centers, and centralized practice units. Appropriate new techniques for communication between the rural practitioner and the referral center should be developed including the application and development of known space technology for communication of laboratory, electrocardiographic, and other diagnostic and evaluative information to the referral center. In addition, payment mechanisms should be perfected to assure that economic barriers will not prevent effective referral and evaluation of patients.

8. *Pre-paid health insurance for rural people.* Every rural resi-

dent must have the costs of medical care assured regardless of personal income or employment status, in order to remove a major economic barrier for patients, practitioners, and institutions that local areas do not have the financial resources to dissolve. Only a comprehensive federally supported national health insurance program can accomplish this.

9. *Training grants for post graduate education.* Federal tax exempt grants for continuing education of physicians and other health personnel in rural practice should be made available both to the practitioners and the medical institutions offering such programs. These could take a variety of forms, but they should offer appropriate and attractive economic incentives to medical and other health professional schools to assure a continuing and responsible role in the postgraduate education of rural practitioners.

10. *Medical school related rural health centers and training clinics.* Incentives should be provided through federal legislation for medical and other health science schools to establish, maintain, and participate in demonstration rural health centers that would provide ambulatory care and training of students, resident physicians, and other trainees in rural primary care situations. The Federal Government should bear the expense for the development, including the building and equipping for such centers and provide staffing arrangements either through PL 91-623 or reimbursement to the schools for professional staffs of these clinics. Increased capitation payments to the schools should be made for all students or trainees who receive part of their training in these satellite rural health centers. Those schools near health manpower shortage areas which decline to participate in such developments should have their capitation payments decreased.

11. *Elimination of matching fund requirements for federal programs in designated rural areas.* Rural areas without financial resources should not be required to provide matching funds for health programs or health related activities. Full federal financing should be provided in such regions and the requirements for matching funds with the concomitant fraud and misrepresentation, eliminated.

12. *Rural health technical assistance mission.* A new rural health technical assistance mission should be developed within HEW and assigned to the Rural Health Bureau to provide direct technical assistance to our own rural areas in all health and health related matters in a manner similar to our technical assistance missions to foreign countries. We should seek and accept World Health Organization participation in such efforts.

13. *Congress should give attention to the 1967 Report by the President's National Advisory Commission on Rural Poverty: The People Left Behind.* The recommendations of this Commission are well-developed, comprehensive, properly focused and should be implemented forthwith.

14. *Establishment of a federally-financed rural network of community health services and health related programs to assure comprehensive health services for all residents in rural areas.* The state and local communities have been and are unable to finance such programs.

15. *A federal rural multi-purpose ombudsman program should be established* rendering direct assistance in health, education, welfare, employment, and other services to rural families throughout the country, and visiting each family at least once a year to assure rural family assistance.

16. *Economic incentives for health institutions* (e.g. medical schools, hospitals, health departments) to involve themselves more directly in the solution of rural health problems, and conversely economic penalties for those which decline to become so involved.

17. Establishment by federal statute of a new civil right to medical care for everyone in an emergency, with appropriate civil and criminal penalties for denial of this right.

18. *Establishment by federal statute of a new civil right to medical care for every sick child,* with appropriate civil and criminal penalties for denial of this right.

19. *Statutory criminal and civil penalties applicable to any public official or employee obstructing, impeding, or delaying any public or private benefit to any person relating to health, education, welfare, or employment.*

20. *Prompt federal action to halt all adverse land use practices*

such as strip mining, uncontrolled timbering, and pollution practices, which are destroying the natural beauty of our rural areas and threaten to make these regions uninhabitable.

21. *Allocation of 1 per cent to 2 per cent of all appropriations for health, welfare, education, and other personal service programs to assure the self-enforcement and delivery of benefits to prospective recipients.* This could finance legal services for assuring availability of services to the beneficiaries.

22. *Allocation of at least 10 per cent of appropriations for categorical health service programs* to permit such programs to assume financial responsibility for diagnosis and treatment of health conditions discovered among their beneficiaries, which are not otherwise within the scope of their programs. The present statute and regulations ordinarily prevent this approach.

23. *Economic, educational, and other incentives for individuals with needed skills to settle and work in rural areas.*

Finally, I would like to restate two recommendations that I made before the United States Senate Subcommittee on Health on March 31, 1971, which warrant repetition.

24. *An amendment to the United States Constitution to guarantee to every adult, responsible for his own support or the support of others, an opportunity for gainful employment consistent with his skills.* The Federal Government should be the employer of last resort. We must stop forcing people to subsidize our economic system through their own unemployment and resulting poverty. There is much productive work needed that can be accomplished throughout the country, including work in the health professions.

25. *An amendment to the United States Constitution to eliminate the present inequality of opportunity* of all kinds for people in the various states by a new definition of "equal protection of the laws," requiring a uniform national standard and full equality nationally in the quantity, quality, and availability of all services and programs related to local, state, or Federal Government. Inequality of opportunity in which government actively participates cannot be eliminated until we adopt a uniform, constitutionally mandated national standard of equality.

I regret the sudden shift from the specific to the global, but the nature of the problems and the legislative process itself unfortunately requires both.

Finally, let me emphasize what I believe is an urgent need to end legislative dabbling and to develop, implement, support, and finance an honest, comprehensive approach to deliver on our promise of equal opportunity for health and the pursuit of happiness.

REFERENCES

1. Health Message from the President of the United States: House Document 92-49, February 18, 1971.
2. Social Security Amendments of 1971: Report of the Committee on Ways and Means on H.R.1, 92nd Congress, 1st Session, House Report No. 92-231, May 26, 1971.
3. Social Security Amendments of 1965: PL 89-97, as amended by PL 90-248.
4. Federal Role in Health: Report of the Committee on Government Operations, U. S. Senate, Subcommittee on Executive Reorganization and Government Research, 91st Congress, 2nd Session, Report No. 91-809, April 30, 1970.
5. National Health Insurance: Brief Outline of Pending Bills, Committee on Finance, U. S. Senate, 92nd Congress, 1st Session, April 26, 1971.
6. S. 3: A Bill to Create a National System of Health Security, U. S. Senate, 92nd Congress, 1st Session, introduced by Senator Edward M. Kennedy, *et al.*, January 25, 1971.
7. S. 1182: A Bill to Establish and Expand Health Maintenance Organizations, U. S. Senate, 92nd Congress, 1st Session, introduced by Senator Jacob Javits, *et al.*, March 10, 1971.
8. A New Life for the Country: The Report of the President's Task Force on Rural Development, March, 1970.
9. Personal Communication: David Z. Morgan, M.D., Assistant Dean, West Virginia University School of Medicine, April, 1971.

SUMMARY AND COMMENTS

Chapter 13

SUMMARY AND REVIEW

DAVID S. HALL

T HROUGHOUT THE CONFERENCE, I was reminded of the story of a seventy-five-year-old man, a rural Appalachian, who decided to marry a girl in her late teens. The old gentleman consulted a physician to seek advice as to how he could be most likely to produce an heir. The embarrassed doctor proposed that, since the wife-to-be was just a girl and might find it "lonely" living with a man of his client's age, the couple should seek a lodger. The guest, the physician suggested, would make the old gentleman's wife cheerful and thus make her more likely to conceive.

Not long afterward, the aged husband returned to his physician and reported: "You were quite right. My wife is pregnant."

After offering his congratulations, the physician cautiously inquired, "And how is the lodger?"

"Fine," the proud gentleman replied, *"she's* pregnant too!"

Not unlike the above gentleman, those who are concerned with producing meaningful and viable solutions to Appalachian or broader rural health problems face major obstacles. In prescribing and arranging the Conference, Drs. Nolan and Schwartz believed that those participating and lodging would not only feel "less lonely" in their various present and future health-related roles but also would contribute to the conceiving and implementing of new solutions to rural health care delivery problems.

A number of comments provide evidence that the Conference did not simply fulfill Ambrose Bierce's definition of "hospitality," which he described as "the virtue which induces us to feed and lodge certain persons who are not in need of food and lodging."[1] Some attended to receive and provide *information,* others perhaps for *confirmation,* each potentially an important contribution. There is always, however, the danger that those who could benefit most from such a conference do not attend, leaving problems and solutions to those concerned and committed persons already aware of the need for resolving what the popular and unpopular media almost universally refer to as the "health crisis."

Although he represented a Social Darwinist view of man which is said not to be accepted today, William Graham Sumner may well have made an important and relevant point in his characterization of what he called "the forgotten man."[2] Simply delineated, "A" (an individual, a group, or collectivity) sees a problem which he thinks needs to be solved. The problem, however, is not "A's" but "X's," although, one might add, that if "A" sees "X's" problem at all, it may be due to the perception that it impinges or may ultimately impinge on "A" himself. "A" and "B" get together (perhaps in a Conference?) and decide that "X" indeed does have a problem. Having identified and agreed upon the problem, "A" and "B" then decide that "C" should take care of "X's" problem, possibly by paying new taxes or through various deprivations, threats, or changes in life style more likely to affect "C" than "A" or "B." To Sumner, then, "C," not "X," is "the forgotten man."

In relation to health phenomena, the issues are obviously more complex. Many of both the "health providers" and the "health consumers" (to use a common false dichotomy, in that we are all consumers of health services and products as well as being, however unwittingly, providers of health) recognize and seek solutions to health care problems, and are thus among the "A's and B's" on questions pertaining to health. A gratifying feature of the Conference and similar ones is that it included among its participants a number of "C's," both providers and consumers of health who, in attempting to meet the goal of alleviating unacceptable rural health conditions, are willing to "pay the price" by, for example, espousing unpopular causes, financial sacrifices, social and professional isolation, modification of previous career activities and plans, and by psychic and other investments in innovative and often precarious approaches.

To continue Sumner's delineation briefly, who is the "X" whose health problems need to be solved or alleviated? The Conference was designed to focus upon the resident of rural Appalachia, hopefully with implications for rural residents throughout the United States, rather than on a particular segment (the aged, the black, the farmer) or anomaly (diabetes or obesity). A few authors tend to confuse "rural" with "agricultural," apparently not recognizing that the vast majority of rural Appalachian residents are not farmers. Beyond this misconception, there is the suggestion, explicit or implicit, in some papers that rural health problems in Appalachia are centered, not exclusively, but primarily in the region's most poverty-stricken residents.

In his excellent and inspiring paper on his experiences with such a population, David Looff correctly notes that ". . . it is the manifold problems of the very poor that are the most vexing." However, I would point to Jerome Schwartz's Chapter, among others, to question Looff's contention that "the stable working class (although they are generally poor by federal income standards), the middle and the upper classes in the region generally succeed remarkably well in providing for their health, education, and welfare needs." Not one of the eight counties described in detail by Schwartz provides (for its general population) health, education, and welfare needs which most of us would find acceptable, not to mention optimal. As he points out, one of the major problems Charles Gilbert faces as a rural dental practitioner is obtaining personal health care for his family and himself. Regardless of his education, occupation, and income, the resident of many rural Appalachian counties simply does not have access to the appropriate range of health care services needed. Thus, I would maintain that, in a very real sense, virtually all of us Appalachian residents are "X's," sharing, however unequally, health problems as a kind of minority group within the larger urban American society.

In his foreword to Matthew Dumont's book, *The Absurd Healer,* Leonard Duhl describes an early experience when, as an intern in Brooklyn, he was called to see a patient in a fifth-floor slum tenement.

> After climbing the stairs with the ambulance attendant and two policemen to protect me, I entered a room which appeared to be no more than twelve feet square. In it were about a dozen people joined

by giant rats circling under the sink and cockroaches on the walls and ceilings. Under the single bulb which lit the room were people preparing food, children playing, couples performing sexual acts, people coughing, smoking—all huddled together in poverty and despair. In the far corner of the room was a woman lying in a pool of blood, having just delivered a baby and the after-birth. Spontaneously, without a thought, I turned to the ambulance driver, perhaps to cover my own anxiety, and asked: "Which one is the patient?"[3]

As with Dr. Duhl, those who have identified health problems as their major career concern soon recognize that a host of anomalies impose themselves upon human beings to a degree that it becomes difficult if not undesirable to identify "the" patient or "the" disease to be treated. The present papers have often painfully and strikingly reinforced an observation first suggested by obstetricians and later expanded by medical sociologists—the concept of a "clustering of pathologies." Physicians first noted the frequency with which congenital anomalies occur in multiple form. As medical sociologist Robert Straus observes, "it is an accepted procedure for a physician who observes an anomaly in a newborn infant to conduct a rigorous examination for other possible signs of defect or malformation, and more often than not these will be found. The 'clustering principle' is seen when trauma affecting one of the major body systems is accompanied or followed by involvement of other systems."[4] Similarly, human social problems tend to cluster together, and many follow or are closely related to medical anomalies, including unemployment, alcoholism, drug addiction, marital disruption, inadequate housing, low income, etc.—"interrelated in a vicious, self-sustaining spiral of despair in which the ability for effective biological, psychological, and social functioning is impaired, cultural isolation increased, and capacity for adaptation to the total environment is destroyed."[4]

A tremendously broad and large if not exhaustive number of health and health-related problems facing rural Appalachia were identified and discussed throughout the papers. (Although the Conference itself was designed so that approximately half the papers presented would focus primarily on problem identification and the other half on proposals of solutions, the latter by no means failed to emphasize the problems at hand, and the former offer at least implicit solutions.)

At this point, a repetitious cataloging of these problems would be of little value. At a general level, perhaps the three single most salient and descriptive terms used in characterizing Appalachia (and to a lesser extent, much of the rural United States) are as follows: *isolation* (geographic, social, and cultural); *poverty* (not of beauty and natural resources but of human capital, of desirable, nonextractive and nonexploitative industry, of a broad range of health, education, and welfare services, and, to some extent, of hope for a better earthly future) ; and *population migration* (movement, often to urban areas outside of Appalachia, of many of the young, healthy, relatively well-educated and employable, leaving behind a population residue with obverse characteristics and without the resources to meet the vast resulting economic and social welfare needs) . This unhappy caricaturization reminds one of Kasper Naegel's statement that although "the truth shall make us free," its discovery and acceptance "shall make us sad, at least for some time."[5]

Despite this melancholy picture, the stance of the contributors is generally not one of despair. For example, David Looff's chapter, "Rural Appalachians and Their Attitudes Toward Health," depicts Eastern Kentucky families as being inner-directed, individualistic, traditional, stoical in manner and speech, fatalistic, and especially fearful of illness. He points to gaps, particularly beyond the infancy period, in the family training patterns of children in the poverty-stricken rural families. Yet, Dr. Looff sees in these families strengths which can be "tapped for redirection." Among the families' potential assets or strengths, he says, are a "person orientation," an "intense feeling-orientation," and a "marked capacity for essentially well-relatedness." Because the family values its solidarity, its fear of illness can be exploited in a positive direction to lead toward acceptance of health services and to reduce the crisis-orientation which characterizes so many recipients of health care in Appalachia.

Viewing the prospects for social change in Appalachia and the rural South, Dr. Looff recommends, "we must start at the beginning of the problem with the very young children," modifying present "fundamental child development patterns which close-in the individual in the lower class, particularly, and make it difficult for many to accept change."

For health professionals in Appalachia, Dr. Looff makes two important observations. First, citing the "therapeutic apathy and nihilistic attitudes" displayed by some health workers, he points out the need for close examination of the professionals' attitudes toward recipients of health care and related services. Second, he stresses that health care planning in rural Appalachia should center upon existing, local agencies with which the population is familiar: "The ultimate success or failure of the various agencies delivering these services to the Appalachian poor depends upon the extent to which each agency can personalize its approach." Ted Hipkins and Leonard Pnakovich both similarly underscore the importance of using as a baseline for expanded services the existing health agencies in the recipients' home locale. On the other hand, Dean Frank W. McKee suggests in his opening remarks that ". . . the planner or those concerned with improving the situation are often better off to start with nothing, than to engage in an attempt to consolidate or abandon outmoded, inadequate, often perilous, but dearly loved institutions. . . ."

Clearly the most controversial paper was Professor William H. Miernyk's "Economic Characteristics of Appalachia and Potentials for Financing Health Care Improvements." Certainly, few disagreed with his opening statements concerning the number and frequent superficiality of journalistic reports assessing the Appalachian economy as failing. (If Appalachia's ratio of health professionals per population is well below the national average, the itinerant reporter per population ratio appears to be quite adequate!)

Considerate disagreement was generated by Professor Miernyk's defense of the expenditure of nearly 80 per cent of the Appalachian Regional Development funds for highway construction rather than for education and health services. As he pointed out, however, this highway development is essentially irreversible and program emphasis will shift to the latter services.

Professor Miernyk presents data which, at least for the broad area and limited time period to which they pertain, show improvement of Appalachia's economic conditions relative to the rest of the nation with the region moving "closer to national averages"* with regard to economic variables such as employment, wages, and income, which, in turn, "should lead to general improvement in basic health conditions." On the other hand, Dr. Schwartz's data on eight contiguous central West Virginia counties present a picture of continued decline in various general welfare indices (as reflected, for example, in a decrease in number of physicians per 100,000 population from 53 in 1960 to 28.4 in 1971). This and other apparent related contradictions suggests, as Schwartz points out, that "Looking at all of Appalachia or at the entire state [of West Virginia] without separating out urban areas from the rural ones or mountain and isolated sections from rural farm areas is a misleading approach." Wide variations within Appalachia are disguised by summary data based on broad political jurisdictions or geographic areas.

Professor Miernyk, in agreement with various other economists, contends that "large parts of rural Appalachia are not economically viable," and that "the best thing that could be done for the people of these subregions is to encourage them to leave." Though recognizing that the urban crisis is associated with ("caused by," he says) migrations of certain rural populations to the cities, Professor Miernyk appears to advocate the Appalachian Regional Commission's "growth point" strategy in which public investments are concentrated in relatively large communities, especially those with considerable growth potential, and are presumably followed by a large rural-to-urban population movement. An important element of the ARC strategy, he emphasizes, is for these population shifts to occur *within* Appalachia rather than from Appalachia to metropolitan areas outside, although it is not clear how migration patterns that have been established during the past three decades will be greatly modified.

---

*Somehow, this conjures up the ludicrous image of the football coach defending his less than happy record by pointing to its increasing similarity to the national average for football coaches.

Thus, it is said, the growth point strategy, with its associated "economies of scale" and positive "external effects," provides sound and realistic directions for Appalachia's future.

We are told that it is *unrealistic* to commit significant direct public investments to enhance rural health care delivery in areas which are not considered "growth points." (It is of little consolation to note that many who dispute the "reality" of rural health solutions also challenge the reality of present expenditures for moon exploration, or for the development of supersonic aircraft for the benefit of a few, or for the transplanting of hearts at an enormous monetary and psychological cost for persons whose life expectancy is increased, at best, for a few months, or to continue the war in Indochina, in part, to "provide for the early and safe return of American prisoners.")

Unless highly objective criteria are developed and implemented for the "politically-free and unbiased" identification and selection of potential "growth points," there is a clear danger of the "self-fulfilling prophesy."[6] That is, if defined as a growth point, however erroneously, and given special attention and funding, a given area is likely to indeed become a growth point.

A second and more disconcerting limitation of the growth point strategy is that it reflects a distinctly urban bias. True, the United States is demographically an "urban nation" (with 73.5% of its residents living in urban places). However, in West Virginia, one of the nation's most rural states, more than six of every ten persons lives in a rural area. Much of the remainder of rural Appalachia is, as Professor Miernyk points out, heavily rural, more particularly "rural nonfarm." Nationally, then, the number of persons living in areas defined by the census as rural total nearly fifty-four million, an incredibly large number of persons to be neglected in favor of more "economical" urban populations and policies. Certainly, a significant number of these 54 million either now live in areas which are accessible to present urban services or to developing growth points. However, as Dr. Abraham Drobny's paper points out, United States definitions of rurality (conventionally limited to areas under 2,500 population, with a few exceptions) may be much too restrictive. The health problems of relatively isolated Appalachian communities with populations between 2,500 to 5,000 or even from 5,000 to 10,000 do not appear to differ greatly from those of many communities clearly defined as rural. Thus, beyond the fifty-four million "officially rural persons" in this country, millions more face health problems which are rural in character. Whatever the actual number, it is too large to be written off in the interests of "economic reality."

Professor Miernyk's paper raises broad issues concerning the degree to which the traditional economic market-place principles are validly reflected in the economics and provision of health care.

Conventional economic principles are not particularly helpful in determining, for example, a) how many physicians are produced (though they are predictive to a greater degree of "who" becomes a physician at all) ; b) physicians' overly frequent specialty choice of the most overcrowded specialty, surgery; c) the practice locations of physicians and other health personnel in areas in which there is already an imbalance of such persons and lesser need and demand for their services than in many rural areas; d) the number, size, and location of hospitals; and e) the commitment of large sums of money to prolong the lives of persons with terminal diseases or the very aged. Unlike most other necessities, health care needs, for the individual, are rather unpredictable and involuntary. Obviously, the consumer is unable to "select" a disease he can afford (frequently, need is inversely related to ability to pay) or a time when he can best pay for needed health goods and services (illness often causing loss or reduction of income and coming at times when income or health insurance coverage are already reduced) . The health client is far from well-informed and sovereign. After he initially seeks care, decisions concerning where, how, when, and from what sources he is treated are usually "technical" and beyond the client's control. Unlike the purchasers of, say, automobiles, health customers or clients (physicians prefer to talk of clientele) are discouraged from "shopping around." They are not guided (or misguided) by advertisements, by health personnel's criticisms of less than highly competent colleagues (competitors) , or by available specifications of the quality and characteristics of needed goods and services. (Even health workers disagree on the criteria to be employed, recognizing that patients and their problems are "individualized" and cannot be easily and meaningfully unitized and standardized.) Relatively few gradations in quality are available; in theory, there are no economy x-ray readings, touring class appendectomies, or second-hand operation rooms (though the patient may have the choice of semi-private or private hospital accommodations or may request, if he is aware of the option, "generic equivalents" to a higher-priced but presumably no more effective brand name drug).

Also often overlooked in accounting for health behavior is that health care, unlike most other goods and services, is frequently not a wanted or pleasurable commodity, because of the anxiety or discomfort and pain often associated with its diagnosis and treatment.

In reality, of course, the choice of seeking no care at all or of visiting only a chiropractor for a suspected malignancy or of limiting one's care to an isolated, technically obsolete general practitioner rather than a highly-trained and reputed specialist is significantly influenced by economic considerations, as are many aspects of health care in general. In fact, in a very real sense, economic factors may be paramount in health care. Although some have argued that the American health system has been ailing for decades (national health insurance was proposed and considered seriously at least as early as 1914,[7] it was not until the economic costs of medical care became seriously inflated that significant changes were widely advocated. It is by now almost a truism to say that inadequacies in the equity, accessibility, and quality of health care are most likely to be recognized when they are reflected in our pocketbooks or in our defense program.

However, as Avedis Donabedian points out, a number of the selected "violations" of classical economic principles briefly mentioned above can also be attributed to institutional spheres outside of the health system, but the peculiarity or uniqueness of health care is that so many of its characteristic properties are not accounted for by accepted economic theories. Donabedian's summary is concise and relevant:

> Briefly, medical care is a service, both necessary and unpredictable,

which must compete with other necessities for which the need is more constantly pressing, or with non-necessities the satisfaction of which is more pleasurable. It must be purchased by a relatively ignorant consumer in a market in which the free operation of consumer choice and the price mechanism are hampered by a variety of restrictive devices. It is, moreover, a service whose receipt or non-receipt by individuals affects society as a whole.[8]

Donabedian's last phrase appears to have particular meaning for Appalachians and many other relatively isolated rural residents who are deprived of the appropriate scope and level of health and related services available to their urban brothers. Even though economic considerations alone may not justify large allocations of funds and personnel resources for health care in areas beyond the fringe of growth centers, it would appear to be both in the public interest and within the realm of public responsibility to commit whatever resources are needed to raise the standards and levels of rural health care. Not only is much of Appalachia (described by Leroy G. Schultz as a "Biafra, American style," a regional "Titicut Follies," the hole in America's sugar-coated donut[9]) a blot on America's landscape, but the health and illness of Appalachia affect much of the entire nation, including many of the urban areas to which Appalachian migrants escape to seek greater equality of opportunity and life style. As Donabedian writes, "Imperfections in the market mechanism for producing and distributing medical care would be more readily tolerated if the benefits of using, and the losses from not using, service were confined to individuals who have made the decision to use or not to use service. As far as medical care is concerned, it is clear that the benefits and losses go beyond the individual and involve others."[10] Appalachian's health care inadequacies represent a threat to the nation, not only by lessening national resources, centering upon economic production, consumption, and national defense, nor by creating greater population migration and consequent urban disruption, but also by reflecting the failure of the broader American society to live up to its promises and potentials.

Dean McKee points out that:

Provision and maintenance of the "good life" for those who live beyond the city limits should have a high national priority, for we are all heavily dependent on these people and the products of their labors. A concerted attack on housing, transportation, poverty, and nutrition, in its larger less medical sense, should have equal stature with health. These highly important items should not be packaged up and foisted off on the health professions as many of our noble leaders seem inclined to do. By the same token, those of us concerned with health problems should not so docilely accept responsibility and castigation for all the ills of society, and should be much noisier in our demands for cooperation from other benefactors, including some politicians, with equally high priority obligations.

These recommendations seem quite sound. Although Schwartz's paper, among others, clearly points out the highly significant interaction between health phenomena and broader societal characteristics, certainly the health profession cannot be charged with the direct responsibility for solving societal problems far beyond the health realm, nor can physicians alone be expected to have the broad level of expertise necessary to modify the present medical system.

Within the narrower perspective of health problems, Appalachia provides a significant message for all health professionals, one reaching far beyond the region's geographic, economic, or political importance. Beyond the Appalachian anomalies for which health institutions are not responsible, the chronic headache (or heartache) of which Appalachia complains is a symptom of illness underlying the larger American health care system. For a variety of reasons made clear in the Conference, Appalachia is "constitutionally" weak and prone to manifest symptoms and signs of illness before they are reflected elsewhere, particularly in urban areas.

Dr. Schwartz's detailed paper on "Rural Health Problems of Isolated Appalachian Counties" provides a careful documentation of many of the limited and declining health and related services and population characteristics in selected, contiguous West Virginia counties. Bemoaning the endless collection of statistics which characterizes much of "the literature" and many conferences, Dr. John Hatch has noted: "experiencing diarrhea in a crowded rural home without toilet facilities is considerably more impressionable than reviewing data on the high rate of intestinal disorder, its probable cause, and the statistical fact that 90 per cent of the housing is dilapidated and without plumbing."[11] Yet, in his paper, and the months of first-hand observation which preceded it, Dr. Schwartz reflects not only a sound and objective understanding of the situations he reports but a strong sense of compassion and concern for the population to which his paper relates. Others less familiar with the lack of current and coherent data characterizing West Virginia may mistakenly misjudge both the difficulty and the value of Dr. Schwartz's useful work.

Dr. David Steinman's paper on "Barriers to Receiving and Delivering Health Care" expresses his interest in and understanding of the historical and contemporary sociocultural factors which enlarge the gap between Appalachian life styles and the delivery of modern health care. Among the most significant contributions of his paper is his identification not only of "attitudinal factors" which affect Appalachian residents' motivation to seek care but also, equally if not more importantly, of "organizational barriers" which hamper such motivation and even block the motivated individual from receiving health services which are indicated. Reporting data from the various surveys and demonstration projects with which he has been identified as a field professor in the University of Kentucky College of Medicine's various outreach programs, Dr. Steinman points out a number of barriers to health care, describes the clustering of pathologies which characterize his study populations, and discusses means of enhancing primary care.

Leslie Dunbar's paper "Human Needs and the American Welfare System," presented during a seemingly wrathful thunderstorm which curtailed electrical power during the Conference, provided its own illumination and provocation. Though it could be misinterpreted as "merely" carefully dissecting and projecting the past, present, and future American welfare system, a topic of interest to but possibly somewhat peripheral from the providers of health care, this thoughtful paper has immediate and direct relevance to the American health care system. Parallels abound. We may ask about the health system, as he asks of the welfare system:

1. Not only "can," but "will" it be made to work more effectively?

2. Can health be made to work while the munitions economy continues?

3. What will happen to it "if peace breaks out?"

4. Can meaningful reform be made to work, "in light of the American practice of well-nigh total irresponsibility for the introduction of new technologies?"

5. What changes will occur in the medical system if we continue and enlarge our tendencies to "contain all of our poor within cities" and retain power in the hands of Congressmen and others who have "not only a lack of concern and sympathy for the poor but manifest antagonism?"

6. Is the health crisis coincidental with "the collapse of our capability to manage large systems" in general?

7. Is the health system, not unlike other large structures, one in which there are few if any "career ladders which reward those who serve the poor well?"

8. Is reform of the medical system likely to be undertaken no more than once in a generation, and what does this mean for present reform notions?

9. Should health care also be federalized, with the government establishing and guaranteeing "costs, benefits, and criteria," without regional differentiation?

10. Is the "mode of financing" really the key issue in health care?

11. Does American medicine "blame the victim" and view the poor as dispensable and not deserving respect?

12. Do rural residents have the right to remain where they are, and is it economical for society to provide health care "where the people are?"

13. How can the ideas, interests, and talents of the poor be recognized and incorporated in the provision of health care?

Dr. Dunbar also calls for, as does Dr. Robert Nolan in his own paper, a "principal of adequacy" for the poor and near-poor, and a "definition and assertion of minimum national standards of health, education, nutrition, housing, etc., below which no individual child or adult would be allowed to fall; and a concomitant translation of such standards into legal rights. . . ."

In a statement that disagrees or goes far beyond Dr. Looff's emphasis upon the need for placing priority on children and modifications of their family rearing patterns, Dr. Dunbar contends:

> . . . there are literally no solutions to American poverty that do not include jobs. To place priority on child welfare appeals to our hearts, and also to our felt need for a beginning point at which to break the cycle of poverty. But I think it will not do, not, at any rate, unless we desire taking a sizable step in the direction of totalitarianism. If not, we shall continue to rely on families for the rearing of children. And the family is held together by a vocation, or vocations. Seen in this respect (and many of the poor do so see it) the current emphasis on children's rights and child welfare can appear as one more sell out, one more double dealing, or at best, one more grotesque irrelevancy, unless accompanied by an equal and prior emphasis on jobs and income.

In short, Dr. Dunbar's excellent paper defies ready summarization. It deserves careful reading and rereading, and thoughtful generalization to the health sphere.

The panel papers by Leonard Pnakovich and Martha Crider represent the deep intensity of thought, concern, and involvement reflected by many consumers as they become actively involved in representing health recipients' interests. Among the health system deficiencies cited by Pnakovich are overutilization of hospitals for diagnosis and treatment, deemphasis of preventive and out-patient care, excessive numbers of surgical procedures, and inadequate cost controls, all of which he traces to the design and operation of health insurance policies. He finds abuses and conflicts of interests in blood bank programs, the provision of eye glasses and other appliances, drug repackaging and prescribing practices, including failure to prescribe generically, chain operations of proprietary hospitals, some of which fail to even provide emergency room services, deemphasis upon health education, and lack of comprehensive care. Advocating a national health insurance plan, Pnakovich points to the positive influence and experiences of the United Mine Workers' Association and its influence on the quality of health care.

In her articulate and impassioned presentation, Martha Ann Crider speaks both as a consumer of health care and one who has seen delivery problems as an executive of Raleigh County, West Virginia's Mountaineer Family Health Plan. Mrs. Crider cites a number of barriers which disadvantage the rural resident who needs health care and, in a vivid analogy, describes how minor preventive measures are recommended when major corrective surgery is indicated. Mrs. Crider questions whether health care is granted the proper national priority, particularly vis-a-vis present emphases on war, defense, foreign aid, and space exploration. Ironically, this country expresses great national concern and devotes untold monies and man-hours to safely recover a child lost in the woods or an adult trapped underground but frequently refuses to devote equal compassion and resources to thousands of less visibly lost or entrapped whose lives could be saved or altered by early diagnosis and treatment of health problems. One is reminded in a painfully real sense that our attitudes toward health sometimes reflect the "military" attitude toward casualties: "one death is a tragedy; ten thousand deaths are a sanitation problem." In a similarly cynical manner, Barbara and John Ehrenreich suggest in *The American Health Empire* that "health is no more a priority of the American health industry than safe, cheap, efficient, pollution-free transportation is a priority of the American automobile industry."[12]

Leslie Falk's "Potential Role of Medical Schools in Improving Health Care Delivery" is critical of present schools of health science. He decries their emphasis upon "super-specialization," "categorized clinics," the "brain drain" and "heart drain" which convert formerly rural students and their wives to "institution-based technologists, the progressive decline of humanitarian attitudes among medical students, and the relative absence of appropriate models of primary care relationships." Dr. Falk sees rural populations, their health problems and broader life styles as underrepresented and misrepresented in medical and related professional schools.

Just as the label "Appalachia" tends to misleadingly homogenize a relatively broad and diverse area, the rubric "rural people," as Falk points out, does not adequately differentiate between those who are mountaineers or plainsmen, rich or poor, with or without a variety of services, etc. In general, though, Appalachian rural people can be accurately characterized as being "poor, educationally disadvantaged and caught in demoralizing vicious circles." Falk emphasizes the rural Appalachian, whose medical care system he sees as having been positively influenced, at least in many areas, first, by the old "check-off" system for coal miners and, since 1949, by the United Mine Workers of American Welfare and Retirement Funds, with its expensive medical care program, including prepaid group practice plans and the original Appalachian Regional Hospital system.

Dr. Falk points to a number of important health demonstrations in Appalachia, including several developed by the Appalachian Regional Commission, the Frontier Nursing Service, home services such as those offered by the Fairmont Clinic and the Family Health Service in Elkins, the Appalachian Regional Hospitals' regional comprehensive health care model, among others.

Although Dr. Falk sees research directed toward rural health care delivery as a highly important function of medical schools, one requiring personnel unlike those presently involved in laboratory or clinical research, he sees most schools as falling far short of their potential and their responsibilities in relation to such research. Falk delineates a number of subject areas requiring investigation which are of particular relevance to medical schools located in or primarily serving rural areas. In addition, he described a number of models of rural health care delivery in which medical schools are or could be involved, including medical student preceptorships with solo medical practitioners, comprehensive community health programs, rural group practices, observation of private family practices, elective rural primary-specialty service, and nurse-focused primary care models.

Among the nation's medical schools, Meharry Medical College stands out not only because of its unique history over nearly a century of training black health professionals but also as a leader in rural health care service activities. At Meharry, Falk and his colleagues have been involved in rural-based delivery programs not only in Tennessee but also as geographically far-ranging as Mississippi, Arkansas, Alabama, and West Virginia. Falk sees a rural field faculty approach as having particular potential.

Looking at broader issues concerning the financing of health services, he sees the proposed Health Maintenance Organizations as significant, providing benefits are clearly comprehensive and there is a ceiling on expenditures. Contrasting the current two basic proposals for National Health Insurance, the Administration's approach of adding Federal monies to the existing delivery system through voluntary health insurance versus the so-called "Kennedy Bill," the Health Security Bill, which is directed toward reorganization of the delivery system, Falk views the latter as offering considerable more potential for rural areas, and presumably for the nation as a whole.

In his discussion of the criteria for a meaningful national health insurance program, Falk refers to the late E. R. Weinerman's conceptualizations, which call for, as counterparts to federal funds for health care, "production and quality control of manpower and facilities," "demonstrations of better methods of training and construction, for experimentation with new types of personnel and facilities." and closer liaison with agencies having such responsibilities. Through incentives for comprehensive prepaid group practice, Falk and Weinerman see greater economy (but not reduced incomes for efficient group practices) and reduction of hospitalization. Also called for are development and financial backing of total health teams to broaden supportive services and payment of full costs of regionalization such as communications and transportation costs of linkages with a range of health resources. In addition, Weinerman advocated other reimbursement schemes, one to encourage group practices by payment of initially higher rates, a second to provide for "quality control and improvement mechanisms such as medical audit by medical peers," and a third to give preference to schools and programs stressing "the primary health team in group practice and regionalization."

If medical schools' potentials extend to the actual roles proposed by Falk, the schools would become "the regional hub" of the health system, sharing with rural communities in the development of rural health care delivery models, not only assuring higher levels of teaching and research but also sharing with rural communities in the development, operation, and evaluation of rural health care delivery models.

In his paper Professor Miernyk says ". . . there has been a tendency in this country to look to federal agencies for means to provide health service to rural areas." This, perhaps, is one of the greatest understatements observed in the papers. Milton Roemer and Abraham Drobny point out in their highly informative papers reasons for this essentially worldwide and by no means recent development. Roemer reviews solutions to rural health care problems attempted around the world, followed by Drobny's relating of Pan American experiences to the solution of rural health problems in the United States. (In referring to the United States in the writing of this summary, I have been tempted to use, for convenience, the adjective "American"; however, this usage is not only ethnocentric and provincial but misleading, in that many of the major, nontechnological innovations in health care delivery have occurred in "American" countries other than the United States.)

Roemer points out that:

> Deficiencies in health services among rural populations are found in every country of the world. In the poorest countries to the richest, in the most agricultural and underdeveloped to the most industrialized and highly developed, the rural population tends to receive a lower level of health service [both qualitative and quantitative] in relation to its needs than the urban.
>
> So long as the economic base of rural medical care depends solely on rural people, deficiencies must persist; agriculture simply has lower per capita productivity and industry. . . . Rural health care can reach the level of urban only by tapping urban wealth.

To reduce the inequities between rural and urban health services, Roemer says:

> . . . almost all countries have undertaken special efforts to compensate for the inherent handicaps of the rural environment. These efforts are nearly always put forth at the national level. It seems to be generally recognized that the solution of rural health care problems must be like the treatment of a systematic disease; the rural symptom is only a manifestation of a systemic disorder, and to alleviate or cure it, actions must be taken to modify the functioning of the total system.

Roemer outlines a number of diverse but often interrelated health actions taken at the national level by central governments, observing striking commonalities of health measures despite great political and economic differences in these countries.

Among these basic measures are the following: a) prevention of disease and promotion of public health measures, especially maternal and child health; b) attracting physicians, whose concentration in large cities is worldwide, to rural areas, both by increasing the overall national supply and by attempting redistribution of physicians through a variety of incentives or requirements; c) the development of ancillary health manpower, ranging from the Russian "feldshers" to the African "dressers"; d) construction of rural hospitals and, more important on a world scale, rural health centers, with diverse staffing patterns; e) enhancement of communication and transportation, the latter said by Roemer to have likely brought greater benefits in rural health care than has enlargement of medical resources in isolated areas; f) quality promotion and maintenance, achieved principally through regionalization; g) increasing economic support, through general revenues, social insurance, programs for special population groups such as migratory or seasonal workers, cooperatives, or national health insurance; h) health service planning and coordination, which Roemer notes, tends to have been launched late in industrialized Western Europe and North America, "where free private enterprise has been so strong."

Some of Dr. Roemer's observations include the following:

> The ultimate solution to rural health care problems . . . is not to be found solely within the borders of rural states or provinces. It demands action on a national level both for mobilization of economic support and for allocation of resources in some proportion to need. Along with these moves, which obviously require governmental initiative, people within a state can organize existing manpower and institutions to be better prepared for national developments, . . . for example, health maintenance organizations, new types of health manpower, and national health insurance.

Dr. Drobny's paper on Pan American experiences and their implications for the United States parallels Roemer's in various respects. Drobny also contends that ". . . health services in the rural areas cannot be self-sustained and autonomous." Although he characterizes Latin American countries as generally more agricultural and more rural than the United States, and facing relatively fewer chronic illness conditions, a number of similarities in health care delivery problems are observed, including an inadequate data base which possibly result in underestimation of rural health problems.

As in much of the rest of the world, the various Latin American approaches are generally based on a regional health service system, centered around an urban core providing a wide range of specialized services and personnel, with outlying satellite facilities offering more primary care, and, in more isolated areas, more minimal health service outposts linked to the intermediate and central service centers. Characteristically, the dependence on auxilliary or ancillary health workers for basic services increases with distance from the urban centers, though provision is made for supervision and referral to higher echelons in the regional system. Mobile units are often utilized in rural communities, though the high maintenance costs and transportation problems associated with the units make them less desirable than permanent structures.

Below the physician level in training and responsibilities, personnel serving health functions range from volunteers in Colombia and Panama advising on health education and related matters to school teachers in Peru giving first aid and elementary health services, to policemen in Chile manning first aid posts.

Dr. Drobny sees striking similarities between the United States and Latin America in the lack of human health resources, especially the relative lack of physicians in rural areas. In this country, he says, ". . . the states and counties either do not have the funds or do not have the interest to provide health services in quality and quantity as needed." Among other common health problems, easier to explain in Latin America than in the United States because of the latter's "enormous technological development," are deficient sanitation, especially provision of potable water, sewage disposal, and garbage collection and treatment.

Latin American experiences in developing and using ancillary personnel to increase physician's productivity and to expand health care capacities are being reflected, in part, in the United States, though without standardization of training, certification, or actual role performance. Among the positions he sees developing in this country are the "physician's assistant," "clinical associate," "nurse physician associate," and the "MEDEX."

Drobny sees potential for the application of the Latin American experiences with regionalized health services, either on a state or county level, ideally with University Medical Centers taking a major role in this development. He also calls for efforts to better utilize existing institutions and legislation to achieve greater coordination and unity in a broad range of social and economic services.

However, Drobny also calls attention to one essential difference between Latin America and the United States. In the former, preventive, therapeutic, and rehabilitative health care services are provided by Ministries of Health or by Social Security Institutions, with private practice being optional for those who desire and can afford it. In the United States, he says, governments below the federal level provide a degree of preventive services, leaving medical care, even for the indigent, as a primarily private endeavor. Without greater federal investment and planning, application of Latin American experiences on a large scale in the United States is problematic.

In his paper on "The Organization of Rural Health Services," T. P. Hipkens calls for greater application of sound management principles for the organization and operation of health services, using, as an example, the Appalachian Regional Hospital system, with its missions of maintaining "good, traditional community hospitals" and "using these hospitals as a baseline for the development of all sorts of innovative and imaginative health and health-related services for the areas they served." He calls for adaption, with modification for health personnel, of the principles of the best rehabilitation facilities: a) the requirement "that the impairment itself be reduced as far as possible"; b) recognition that with the severely handicapped one must also work at reducing all of the obstacles to optimum function," focusing on the total handicap; c) "conditions and staff attitudes must be fostered to insure that the impairment reduction and total handicap approach has the possible chance," a therapeutic climate; and d) building "a mechanism for follow-up in the best sense," continuing and complete. The principles, he says, are best transferable into health under the "levels of care" concept (which recognizes intensive care, intermediate, extended, home, ambulant, and self-care).

After tracing the application of these principles with the Appalachian Regional Hospital system, Hipkins proposed some general rules: a) there are no pat answers; b) build no more hospital beds, developing other alternative, more appropriate levels of care; c) proliferate the new services from an established baseline; d) be willing to be an enabler or catalyst or facilitator, e) give proper organizational status to all levels of care; f) provide equitable rewards to "other" levels of care workers; g) with opposition, look for "soft spots"; h) consider the program manager concept; and i) develop an understandable and explainable concept (for staff, trustees, community).

Among the organizations represented which are reflective of the current concern with so-called "consumer representation" or "participatory democracy" is the Health Education Advisory Team (HEAT) serving Marion County, West Virginia. As Joan White points out in her paper, the mission of HEAT is to "provide an improved health care delivery system to all consumers in Marion County, especially those in the lower income bracket and to insure that these consumers are aware of the benefits available to them through the HEAT program." As Mrs. White says, "traditionally, responsibility for the development of health services rested with the providers of medical care." Even among the various providers who are concerned with and aware of the need for health programs reflecting consumer's needs and interests, misinterpretation often results, one factor being that consumers who utilize health services, and with whom providers are at least partially familiar, are by no means necessarily reflective of a given area's entire population. To help counteract this and related misinterpretations of consumers, HEAT is attempting to "sensitize the broader community to health problems and stimulate involvement in the search for solutions, to promote a positive partnership between the health consumer and the health provider, to provide consumer groups with the tools of effective participation, and to cooperate with health institutions in developing a constructive working relationship with consumers."

As a discussant of the Roemer and Hipkens papers, Robert Eakin describes the application at the Elkins-based Family Health Service of a number of the international solutions to rural care delivery identified by Roemer. The Family Health Service is "designed to bring about 20,000 disadvantaged rural people into the mainstream to comprehensive health services by eliminating barriers thereto of ignorance, timidity, lack of transportation, and lack of adequate financial resources, starting within the framework of a highly developed multi-specialty group practice, a general and a convalescent hospital." Among the rural problems cited by Roemer with which the home-care-oriented Family Health Service seems particularly suited to contend are those of attracting physicians and retaining them in rural areas, providing economic support for health services, and to a lesser degree, transportation. Eakin believes that the group practice nucleus is attractive to physicians and offers valuable professional relationships and financial security not necessarily found in solo practices or small partnerships. With regard to economic support, the Family Health Service and its participants, 6,400 of an estimated 8,800 eligible families, are fortunate in having available federal funds provided on "a last dollar concept" for the provision of health care. The importance of this special economic support is indicated by the statistic showing that the Family Health Funds are currently paying 72.5 per cent of the members' health costs, the families and third parties paying the balance. Attempts to reduce transportation barriers are being made through the provision, at low, scaled costs to the users, of two health vans to transport patients to health care providers through daily scheduled routes.

Helen L. Johnston begins her insightful, incisive, and one might even say "appropriately incensed" discussion with a question: "Is rural United States really an 'underdeveloped country?' " Pointing to Dr. Roemer's review of the massive rural health measures undertaken and improvement achieved throughout the world by various countries, many, the objects of foreign aid and technical assistance from the United States, she asks "Is it possible that we need some foreign aid and technical assistance *in reverse* to help us solve our rural health problems?" She proposes that we need to ask why these countries grant such high priority to health measures, suggesting that it reflects recognition that sound bodies and minds are soundly economic, productive workers being healthy and healthy countries being productive. She also questions the economics and sense of values reflected in the notion that health services be developed only in "growth centers."

Faced with comparative indices such as infant mortality rates which show the United States lagging behind many so-called "less developed nations," many trace the unfavorable position of the United States to its large population and its heterogeneity, citing especially the pockets of minority groups—among others, Indians, blacks, inner city ghetto residents, Appalachian and isolated rural residents. Yet, the population density of the United States is comparatively low, a number of other countries with equal or higher health status indicators are far from homogeneous, and the growth center concept essentially overlooks many of the population groups where health problems are most pronounced if infrequently enunciated.

In an ironical account, Mrs. Johnston describes a rural health care delivery model attempted by the Farm Security Administration nearly a generation ago. Incorporating "outreach workers," capitation payment for health care, small group practices, consumer participation, and negotiated arrangements with physicians, all of which sound very contemporary and are among present solutions discussed, the F.S.A. approach was terminated by Congress as "too radical." At the moment, similar development labeled "health maintenance organizations" are accepted as conservative, as Mrs. Johnson points out.

She discusses in her paper the disparity between "the community of the problem" and the "community of the solution." As with the contributors in general, she sees the "real solutions" to health problems not by a single community in isolation but by a linkage of communities or, as in the foreign countries described in the papers, in the nation as a whole.

The paper "Model Health Care Delivery Systems," by Murray B. Hunter describes the Fairmont (Marion County, West Virginia) clinic and its two satellite offices, a group practice providing comprehensive health services to rural and "semi-rural" people. Historically, the character of the clinic and its relationships with its major clientele, coal miners and their families, may be traced to the earlier check-off arrangements and medical care grievance committees characteristic of many mining communities as well as to financial support of the United Mine Workers of America Welfare and Retirement Fund. Staffed by salaried physicians, the three clinic offices reflect, Hunter says, the "traditional one-to-one doctor-patient encounter" model, with "health center trappings (social work, physical therapy, pharmacy service, ancillary support, visiting specialists)."

Dr. Hunter views this form of health care delivery as economical, given an accounting system other than the fee-for-service method, but does not support the substitution of nurse practitioners or physician assistants or related ancillaries for the general physicians providing primary service.

Given the regional topography, Dr. Hunter finds it desirable and feasible to locate satellite offices up to a radius of about thirty miles from the central clinic, though he does acknowledge a difficulty of information transfer from one location to another when health care for a given patient is shared by both a satellite and a central clinic.

Though favoring salaried arrangements, Dr. Hunter suggests that varied arrangements with fee practice physicians desiring supportive relationships with a clinic (e.g. home health, pharmacy, laboratory, or transportation services or consultations) are possible and might serve to reduce the isolation of solo physicians.

Dr. Hunter is not optimistic concerning the ease with which rural group practices may be developed, pointing to various difficulties as well as to opposition of local vested interests.

Offering "political advice" to rural people, Dr. Hunter urges that, as a condition for federal support, HMO's be completed to "redress the maldistribution of medical services" by assuming responsibility for providing health care for a underserviced population segment, either rural residents or inner city ghetto dwellers. "It is time," he says, "that federal monies were used to create social change rather than, as under Medicare, buttress existing ways of doing things." He adds that "we do need help in the form of rational federal legislation in which logic shall reign rather than vested interest. New legislation should interfere with medical practice and should not underwrite the *status quo*."

Dr. Hunter also joints Dr. Falk, among others, in assessing the achievements of medical schools as falling short, reflecting models antithetical to good practice and treating community or rural clinic practice models as electives rather than providing institutionalized expectations and experiences. In addition, he supports proposals also advanced by Drs. Dunbar and Nolan for guaranteed availability of an acceptable level of modern medical care for all Americans.

In her paper, "The Family Nurse and Primary Health Care in Rural Areas," Gertrude Isaacs describes the relatively new concept in this country of the "family nurse" as a provider of primary health care from the perspective of the Frontier Nursing Service's forty-six years of experience with this approach. Forming the nucleus of the F.N.S., which serves southeastern Kentucky's Leslie County and parts of Perry and Clay Counties, the family nurse is a registered nurse with special preparation.

Dr. Isaacs describes a number of advantages of the family nurse (or nurse-midwife). The nurse-midwife's basic skills, extended by one year of additional training in diagnosis and management of common health problems, permit her to extend services to the entire family economically, leaving the physician to perform tasks requiring greater training. Rural manpower problems are reduced because nurses are in much greater supply than physicians and are geographically more equitably distributed. A frequently unrecognized advantage is that the nurse has traditionally been trained to perform more nurturant or expressive roles, a quality of considerable importance to many isolated residents, while the physician is more involved in instrumental or curative roles in which the nurse, by training, is less well-suited.

Dr. Isaacs characterized the F.N.S. as a series of strategically situated, moderately equipped nursing outposts, primary health centers from which no family served in more than an hour's travel time. Each outpost is accessible to the hospital or health center, where a resident physician is available and where further referral may be arranged as needed.

Outpost nurses diagnose and manage common health problems, provide prenatal, postpartal, and healthy-child care, family planning, and, when necessary, home delivery, combining treatment, prevention, and health maintenance skills. Outposts are visited regularly by a physician and a utilization review committee, a field nursing supervisor, and a coordinating nurse.

At the hospital, patients are screened by a nurse and greater supportive and diagnostic facilities and services are available, in addition to a physician for additional consultation or referral if indicated.

Uncomplicated maternity care is provided by the nurse-midwives who perform approximately 95 per cent of the deliveries.

The original F.N.S., started by Mrs. Mary Breckinridge, was based on an extensive survey of local citizens and their problems and wants. Dr. Isaacs stresses the long-established pattern of local citizen participation as being still crucial to the success of the F.N.S.

The more recent indigenous health worker concept reflected in many OEO projects has not emerged at the F.N.S. However, Dr. Isaacs makes the highly interesting observation that because individuals are beginning to expect remuneration for taking care of an ill family member (and low birth rates and migration are reducing availability of persons for such services), the establishment of new patterns will be necessary.

Dr. Isaacs sees the introduction of family health workers as premature, suggesting this would only add to confusion "until the areas of responsibility for primary health care provided by the family nurse have been more clearly defined and legal sanction established . . ." Given the forty-six years of experience by the

F.N.S. with the family nurse, and the apparent success of and enthusiasm for the program, one might expect somewhat greater confidence in the exploration of new roles and relationships for additional types of health manpower.

In projecting the future of the F.N.S. and other relatively small agencies providing primary health care, Dr. Isaacs describes a dilemma. Competition with larger agencies for federal funding appears to be crucial to the viability of such agencies. Yet, many complain, the recommendations or requirements of federal, state, and regional agencies are seen as costly (in time, effort, and money), as sometimes unrealistic, and as threating to local autonomy. Dr. Isaacs suggests that the solutions to health problems associated with isolation and poverty "require a system with a higher degree of ingenuity, adaptability, and flexibility that are based on a knowledge of the area, its people, and its resources. Furthermore, Dr. Isaacs contends that the larger, more highly organized agencies that are more able to willingly meet bureaucratic rules and regulations, and thus receive funding, are alien, less individualized and relatively impersonal, thus not acceptable, except in dire emergencies, to the mountaineer needing health services.

On the other hand, many would argue, there is a clear need for broad-scale regional health planning, avoiding duplication of effort and the proliferation of unrelated agencies, and expanding the "community of solutions" to a regional, state, or federal level, achieving economies of scale, uniform and equitable levels of care, and coordinated regional health care delivery patterns. One of the important unanswered questions of these papers relates to the issue of achieving an optimal relationship between *local* perceptions of health care needs, values, wants and solutions, and *regional, state,* or *federal* determinations (with meaningful authority and power) of health priorities, comprehensive health plans, quality standards, economic support mechanisms, manpower projections, training programs, and distributional criteria, construction of health facilities, and many other related elements of the health system which have previously emerged with relatively little conscious planning and rationality, or when planned, have too often been designed to benefit particular vested interests rather than the broader society.

Dr. Robert L. Nolan's paper, "Federal Action Needed for Rural Health," captures, perhaps more than any other single paper, the stance and conclusions of the participants with regard to the solutions of Appalachian and broader rural health problems in the United States.

"As a noneconomist," he says, "I personally can see no substantial improvement in rural health conditions without massive federal assistance."

Dr. Nolan views the solutions to lie significantly with the Federal Government through broad-scale legislation accompanied by sound and imaginative implementation and enforcement. He emphasizes that: "ultimately, legislative action that is designed to permanently improve health and the quality of life in rural areas must be the product of a public policy committed to deal comprehensively with such issues."

In the meantime, though such a comprehensive commitment is still lacking, for reasons openly faced in Dr. Dunbar's paper, a variety of recent or planned federal legislation bearing upon health offers potential for meaningful solutions.

One imposing fault noted by Dr. Nolan is the multiplicity of uncoordinated, uncorrelated federal health programs (administered in twenty-four separate departments and agencies), many of which are characterized at present by sudden, inconsistent policy changes and rapid personnel turnover, especially at key administrative levels. (Receiving few laughs was a recent "joke line" passing through government health agencies: "If the boss calls, find out his name!")

The several dozen health manpower training programs designed to increase the number of health personnel through grants and loans to trainees or funds to education institutions have succeeded, Dr. Nolan suggests, in increasing total supply, the expenditures of these federal monies have not been effective in offering incentives for the resulting personnel to locate in areas with the greatest health manpower shortages. Neither the President's more recent proposals to forgive loans for medical school graduates nor the new family practice training program, or programs for other health professional categories, appears to be a realistic solution to the health manpower shortage in rural areas.

Other federal program obstacles are the narrowness of various categorical efforts (e.g. milk for school children) and, of particular concern to rural and depressed areas, the need for matching funds from local areas with highly limited resources (as required, for example, by health demonstration programs under the Appalachian Regional Development Act of 1965 and by health facilities construction programs ranging from Hill-Burton to the Federal Housing Administration). Even when monies for construction of rural hospitals and other facilities are obtained, often at considerable sacrifice, many rural facilities remain empty or partially used because of staffing problems.

Federal payment of health services under Medicare and Medicaid programs and a variety of other federal programs have had the effect, Dr. Nolan points out, of reinforcing existing limitations of the health system. Medicare, for example, has given the rural elderly a payment mechanism but not a network of accessible services.

Some of the various national health insurance proposals would presumably extend rural services. However, it is pointed out that "financing mechanisms have thus far favored urban areas where there is a concentration of population, facilities and employee groups."

Noting the apparent inadequacies of various federal health and related programs makes even more striking and disconcerting the observation that many rural residents (due to their remoteness from agencies and lack of information about and experience with such agencies) are unable to or have great difficulty receiving even the limited benefits of federal programs for which they are eligible.

A substantial portion of Dr. Nolan's paper is devoted to some twenty-five legislative and policy steps which he proposes to "translate the current rhetoric into meaningful action." Least surprising, given Dr. Nolan's early and sustained involvement in the Emergency Health Personnel Act of 1970 (PL 91-623) is his call for "early innovative and imaginative implementation of this new law," with flexible program units located near the inner city and rural problem areas.

Most of his proposals are focused distinctly or primarily on rural health (e.g. establishment of a major Rural Health Bureau with the Department of Health, Education and Welfare, to which a new rural health technical assistance mission should be developed; and, in keeping with his previous discussion, elimination of matching fund requirements for health programs in designated rural areas). Others also relate directly to health care but are relevant to the larger population, urban and rural (e.g. establishment by federal statute of a new civil right to medical care for every sick child, and similarly, for everyone in an emergency, with appropriate civil and criminal penalties for denial of these rights). Still other proposals relate less directly to health but are of obvious relevance (e.g. for economic and other incentives for individuals with needed skills to settle and work in rural areas; and prompt federal action to halt adverse land use practices such as strip mining, uncontrolled timbering, and pollution, which are destroying the beauty and threatening the inhabitability of rural areas).

More drastically, and at a more global level, Dr. Nolan calls for two amendments to the United States Constitution:

1. "To guarantee to every adult responsible for his own support or the support of others an opportunity for gainful employment consistent with his skills," with the Federal Government "the employer of last resort." (This proposal, of course, it likely to be challenged by persons of quite different political and economic persuasions, including perhaps a small but growing number who challenge the validity of the assumption that all "able and responsible" working-age adults (or even males) should be gainfully employed.)

2. "To eliminate the present inequality of opportunity of all kinds for people in the various states by a new definition of 'equal protection of the laws,' requiring a uniform national standard and full equality nationally in the availability of all

services and programs related to local, state, or Federal Government."

The preceding Conference paper presented was "What It Would Take for Me to Practice in an Isolated Rural County," by William Taylor Fithian III, a fourth-year medical student at West Virginia University's School of Medicine. Recognizing and personally applauding the values which Dr. Fithian reflects, I found myself hoping that he is representative of other rural Appalachian students and that he, and they, will indeed find positive enticements to practice—not rural medicine but modern medicine in rural settings. Throughout his presentation, as the intriguing drama of whether one William Taylor Fithian III will locate in Letter Gap or River City or Megalopolis unfolded, one sensed that the presenter himself was undergoing an intensive self-examination (perhaps due, in part, as an earlier paper decried, to his lack of exposure to health care in rural areas in his institutionalized medical school experiences), and that the story itself would not be concluded that day, but must await the writer's decision as to an appropriate conclusion.

Dr. Fithian expects the community in which he elects to locate to meet certain criteria with regard to four fundamental elements:

1. Family considerations (e.g. opportunities for his wife's career; and access to libraries, theaters, and related "cultural" activities, either in or accessible to the selected community.

2. Community involvement, e.g. health priorities; attitudes toward the natural environment and toward the alleviation of poverty); educational climate—limited educational facilities and curricula being frequently cited as major barriers to the location of professionals and of new industries in Appalachia.

3. The professional (health) community (e.g. having more than a single physician as well as including a health team of dentists, nurses, social workers, pharmacists and other paramedical personnel; and adequate hospitals and clinics.

4. Access to a major medical center (not merely one physically accessible but one open to and supportive of private physicians in a remote rural area).

In a tentative conclusion, Dr. Fithian suggests that an acceptable rural location might be identified, but that, without changes, both in a community and outside, he would be precluded from a more or less permanent practice within the initial community and would perhaps become a transient physician.

Surprisingly, the papers devoted comparatively little attention to discussion of national health insurance, whose arrival in the near future seems inevitable. On the other hand, national health insurance programs were proposed and considered seriously at least as early as 1914 and legislation for national health insurance has been introduced in every session of the Congress since 1943. Moreover, much of the present emphasis on such insurance is centered around the determination of a financial mechanism to extend health care to more people rather than to enhance the accessibility, equity, comprehensiveness, and continuity of health care delivery. Among the criticisms of most presently proposed schemes are reinforcement of the present fee-for-service system, said to be uneconomical and inefficient; dependence on private health insurance companies, who are charged with responsibility for many of the present inadequacies; lack of viable mechanisms for controlling soaring costs; regressive taxation for support of insurance coverage; and limited consumer and community participation in program planning.

None of the papers advocates "merely" pouring more money into health care without otherwise modifying the health care delivery system. Increasingly, it is recognized that the nations whose health eggs are generally placed in a national health insurance or health service basket spend less, both absolutely and relatively, on health care than the United States. (Sweden, for example, spends about 5 per cent of its gross national product on health care, roughly 71 per cent of our rate, while Great Britain devotes only 4 per cent, 57 per cent of the United States rate.) [13]

Health manpower problems attracted particular attention, particularly the decline in available physician services. Although, contrary to popular opinion, the actual ratio of physicians to general population is increasing, not decreasing (in the United States, the number of medical doctors has grown nearly 25 per cent faster than the total general population over the last two decades) ,[14] as many as one-third of the "new physicians" now devote their time primarily to activities other than direct patient care (e.g. research, administration, teaching, and public health). Specialization has taken a further toll in the availability of physicians for primary care. As a number of papers made apparent, the physician shortage is particularly acute in rural areas, Appalachia in particular.

Quite possibly, the situation may be even more serious than is realized, for many areas of the United States are becoming dependent on physician's services on an influx of foreign medical graduates (FMGs). Nearly 15 per cent of all the nation's physicians are FMGs, and, at present, the FMGs represent nearly 20 per cent of all new licentiates in the United States and more than one of every four hospital house officers.[15]

My ongoing and incomplete survey of new members of the West Virginia Medical Association (from 1961 to 1970) shows that 142 (34.1%) of the total of 417 new members are FMGs. In the first seven years, 18 per cent of the medical population surveyed were foreign graduates but from 1968 to 1970, as many as 54 per cent were FMGs, and from January to May, 1971, as many as 77 per cent were FMGs.

These observations do not represent a "xenophobic Appalachian reaction" to "outsiders," although the few sound evaluations of the quality of FMG's medical training and practices have not adequately eliminated English language biases in examinations conducted by the Educational Council for Foreign Medical Graduates nor the perhaps ethnocentric assumption that "American" medical education (United States and Canadian) provides superior preparation for medical practice in the United States. On ECFMG examinations passed by 98 per cent of United States medical school graduates, only 40 per cent of FMGs achieve a passing score, and one-fourth who pass achieve the minimal passing score of 75, and an additional one-fourth score from 76-79.[16]

Most FMGs are required to serve a year or more of an internshop, but this, Dr. Harold Margulies has suggested, cannot be expected to erase deficiencies of foreign medical education. Long ago, he points out, we "abandoned the system under which physicians were allowed to practice medicine following apprenticeships if they could pass the tests for licensure. In the case of foreign medical graduates, we have virtually reverted to that obsolete device. Inadvertently, we in the United States have established two standards of medical practice.[17] To the extent the rural areas become increasingly dependent on FMGs, this problem demands closer examination in relation to health manpower deficiencies.

Among the most commonly advocated remedies of the health care problems, the manpower problem in particular, are expansion of the number of both "conventional" and "new" types of health providers. In general, these proposals assume, J. Thomas May observes in an interesting communication:

> Only the conventionally-trained health professionals (physicians, nurses, etc.) are legitimate distributors since they alone are adequately prepared for the work. The innovations which have been suggested, such as the MEDEX and the various levels of assistants and aides, are simply attempts to define particular tasks and areas of work *within* the traditional hierarchy. . . . The rationale which is often used for these 'para-professionals' is instructive—they will "free the physician" of menial tasks and increase the "efficiency of the team."[18]

Decrying the lack of new input from health consumers, other than a "certain paternalism" in relation to advice in administrative details, he suggests that "the controlling assumption in all of the evaluations of the "crisis" appears to be that there is no correct form of health care, that it is based on conventional health professionals, and that all people want it."[18]

Others have pointed out that manpower proposals neglect to provide avenues for upward mobility (in which, for example, a successful nurse may become a physician without "starting all over again"), and tend to center on "feminine roles" (with corresponding subordination, economic limitations, rigid work hours, etc.). New manpower roles are developed without adequate recognition of deficiencies which, in part, account for the shortage of active nurses despite there being some 500,000 to 600,000 inactive qualified nurses in the United States.[19] This is not necessarily to imply that the new manpower should be drawn from this pool of nurses, but to suggest that the factors which lead nurses to become inactive be considered and reduced in new manpower schemes.

In 1948, Milton I. Roemer and Frederic D. Mott completed *Rural Health and Medical Care,** which has become one of the classics in its field. Reexamining this book (shelved, oddly enough, in the library's "old books section") after reading the above papers, I found myself experiencing a deja vu. Writing nearly a quarter-century ago, Mott and Roemer not only described and documented many of the same persistent rural medical problems described here, but they also called attention to recognition of the special rural social problems dating back to an 1862 report submitted to President Lincoln by a Dr. W. W. Hall.†

Nearly a quarter-century ago, the authors saw health insurance as having been accepted, saying "the issue today is whether health insurance should be voluntary or compulsory, whether it should be sponsored entirely by independent private groups or by the Federal Government on a nationwide basis."‡ In addition, they pointed out that "to claim the voluntary health insurance plans can solve the overwhelming problem of medical costs, as is done by certain particular groups, is simply not to face economic facts or the lessons of worldwide as well as American experience."* The "contemporary" health insurance debates, in the United States, then, are as "modern" as the late 1940's.

Similarly, Mott and Roemer noted that "happily for the rural population, today's planning for improved health facilities is based largely on the concept of regionalization."† Today, the banner of regionalization is being waved once again.

The authors' identification of "cultural lag" as a particularly useful concept in understanding and predicting rural problems seems, if anything, even more relevant today. As they explain technological changes or scientific "advances" tend to occur considerably more rapidly than the changes in attitudes and social organization necessary to make adjustments to the changes. As the above papers have demonstrated, the differential or lag is more extreme in rural areas.

---

*Mott, Frederick D. and Roemer, Milton, I.: *Rural Health and Medical Care*. New York, McGraw-Hill, 1948.

†*Ibid.*, p. vi.

‡*Ibid.*, p. 480.

Ibid., p. 481.

†*Ibid.*, p. 499.

A number of the present papers call for additional research focusing upon health care delivery. There is increasing recognition of the need for devoting a larger segment of the health research dollar to social organizational phenomena impinging against effective and equitable health care delivery rather than to narrow technological foci in which knowledge, however inadequate, has essentially outrun the former. Moreover, less than 3 per cent of the national health expenditures are allotted to *all* health research and development, an appalling 7 dollars per man, woman, and child, *versus* per capita costs of 30 dollars for space exploration, and 525 for war and national defense efforts.[20] No other major American industry spends so small a proportion of its resources on evaluation of its goods and services and on improvements of its product and delivery systems.

An old Yiddish proverb suggests: "one fool can ask more questions than ten sages can answer." The above papers reflect considerable wisdom, both in their identification of rural health problems and in the discussion of present and projected programs for the partial solution of these problems. However, as Professor Isidore S. Falk observes in his 1971 Michael M. Davis Lecture:

> We are in trouble with respect to medical care not so much because we have failed to recognize existing needs or to anticipate prospective inadequacies, but more because we have lacked the courage and determination to take needed action over the resistance of those who were content with current practices or who fear change. Again and again, we have identified goals and declared good intentions, but we have stultified many of our undertakings through shackling compromises.[21]

Subsequent conferences and research need to be focused not only upon a variety of health care delivery alternatives but also upon the identification of barriers and means of reducing obstacles to modification of the health care delivery systems.

REFERENCES

1. Bierce, Ambrose: *The Devil's Dictionary.* Mount Vernon, New York, Peter Pauper Press, 1958, p. 29.
2. Sumner, William Graham: The Forgotten Man, in Albert Galloway Keller and Maurice R. Davie (Eds.): *Essays of William Graham Sumner.* New Haven, Yale University Press, 1934, Vol. 1, pp. 466-96.

3. Duhl, Leonard J.: Foreword to Matthew P. Dumont: *The Absurd Healer: Perspectives of a Community Psychiatrist.* New York, Science House, 1968, pp. 11-12.

4. Straus, Robert: Social Change and the Rehabilitation Concept, Ch. 1 in M. P. Sussman (Ed.) : *Sociology and Rehabilitation.* Washington, American Sociological Association, 1965, p. 2. See also his valuable related article, Poverty as an obstacle to health progress in our rural areas, *Am J Public Health, 55:*1772-79, 1965.

5. Naegel, Kaspar: Elaine Cumming (Ed.) : *Health and Healing.* San Francisco, Jossey-Bass, Inc., 1970, p. 53.

6. Merton, Robert K.: *Social Theory and Social Structure.* (rev. and enlarged ed.) Glencoe, Ill., Free Press, 1957, pp. 421-36.

7. Harris, Richard: The annals of legislation: Medicare, *The New Yorker,* Vol. 42, July 2, 1966, pp. 26-62; Editors of *Fortune: Our Ailing Medical System.* New York, Perennial Library, 1970.

8. Donabedian, Avedis: Social responsibility for personal health services: An examination of basic values. *Inquiry,* Vol. 8 June, 1971, p. 18.

9. Schultz, Leroy G.: Rural America: Our gross national product, *Iowa J Social Work,* Vol. 3, 1970, p. 48.

10. Donabedian, Avedis: Social responsibility for personal health services: An examination of basic values. *Inquiry,* Vol. 8, June, 1971, p. 16.

11. Hatch, John W.: Discussion of the "how" of community participation in delivering health care, *Bull N Y Acad Med, 46:*1985, 1970.

12. Health Policy Advisory Center: *The American Health Empire: Power, Profits, and Politics.* New York, Vintage Books, 1971, p. vi.

13. Editors of *Fortune* op. cit., p. 38.

14. Ibid., p. 44.

15. Ibid., p. 45.

16. Panel on Foreign Medical Graduates: *Report of the National Advisory Commission on Health Manpower.* Vol. 2, U.S. Government Printing Office, Washington, D.C., 1967, pp. 96-97.

17. Margulies, Harold: The foreign medical graduate and the United States. *J Med Ed,* Vol. 41, Part 2, Sept., 1966, p. 251.

18. May, J. Thomas: Communication: The history of medicine and the "crisis" in medicine, *Inquiry,* Vol. 8, June, 1970, p. 63.

19. Editors of *Fortune,* op. cit., p. 53.

20. DeBakey, Michael E. and Lois: Medical research is hurting, *Saturday Review,* Vol. 54, Oct. 16, 1971, p. 70.

21. Falk, I. S.: National Policies and Programs for the Financing of Medical Care, Center for Health Administration Studies, Graduate School of Business, Univ. of Chicago, 1971.

PROBLEMS OF PROVIDING DENTAL CARE IN ISOLATED RURAL AREAS

CHARLES B. GILBERT

T HERE ARE some definite advantages and disadvantages to living and practicing dentistry in a small town or rural area.

It is nice to be able to let your children play or go to school without worrying about them being molested or bothered by the criminal element that is so prevelant in the cities today. Air pollution is not a problem in most rural areas. It is an advantage for the recent graduate to start a practice with more than enough patients to keep busy. It seems, too, that the income is greater in the first four or five years in a rural area. This tends to level out, however, and our urban counterpart catches up with us in about five years. After about five years the urban practice seems to be in a better financial situation. I feel that the competent dentist can make a good living in the city or rural area.

However, one problem that really concerns me is the lack of medical facilities and personnel to meet the requirements of my family. I am so far from adequate medical care that it frightens me sometimes. I am approximately thirty miles from the nearest physician and about sixty miles from our pediatrician. Thirty to fifty miles is not far, if you have good roads, but in my area, thirty miles means about one hour of travel time. My daughter requires treatment for allergies. This means a trip to Charleston routinely. Every few weeks we must take an entire day to see the allergy specialist for just twenty minutes. On our last visit to Charleston, for example, we left Glenville at about 6:00 AM and returned home at 4:00 PM. I often wonder what I would do in case of a real medical emergency.

Furthermore, in a rural area it seems that the school system usually suffers. We do not have an elementary school in Glenville;

my daughter must be transported about fifteen miles. I was very apprehensive when my six-year-old daughter boarded a school bus for her first year of school.

We have a high school, but it too suffers. Lack of qualified teachers is a problem in most rural areas, but not quite so severe in Glenville. With Glenville State College located there, we seem to have more qualified teachers available than most places. However, apathy of the people in the community and lack of funds add up to many problems. Most of the residents in Gilmer County are elderly people whose children have grown up and left the area. Therefore, it is most difficult to get them to support any issue to improve our schools. Why should they vote for a bond issue that might raise their taxes? After all, it really does not concern them now.

Poverty is a very real problem in the rural areas. I have many patients living in substandard housing. Many do not have enough food to satisfy their basic needs. Most of these people seem to have accepted this as their lot in life and never try very hard to change it.

Professional and social isolation is a very real concern for me. I have seen other practitioners who have gone to rural areas and never did a thing to keep up with new techniques or materials. They do not pursue postgraduate education. After a few years they become so stagnant that it is really frightening. I personally do not want to end up this way.

Recreation, religious activity, and social life are rather limited in a rural area. Recreation in Glenville is a definite problem for our young people. My family does not suffer in this respect since we enjoy outdoor activities. We have a small farm out in the country and spend most of our free time there; in other words, we create our own recreational activities. If we want to see a good movie or concert, the situation changes a little. Our nearest movie theater is about fifty miles away. More often we have to travel farther to see movies suitable for a family. Many times we travel as far as Charleston or Morgantown, 90 and 115 miles, respectively, from Glenville.

I am the only full-time practicing dentist in my county. One adjacent county, Calhoun, does not have a dentist. Gilmer County has about 8,000 people and Calhoun County has about 7,000 people. I also have patients coming from other counties. The American Dental Association suggests a dentist-patient ratio of one dentist to 2,500 patients is near ideal. As you can see, I am supposed to provide dental care for nearly seven times that many people. If I am not careful, I end up providing only emergency care and neglecting preventive care. This, of course, is not fair for the patients really concerned about dental care.

In other words, I must be prepared to work longer hours, accept more responsibility, deprive my family of adequate medical care, and accept lower fees for dental treatment—just for the privilege of practicing dentistry in a rural area.

THE ORGANIZATION OF RURAL
HEALTH SERVICES

Theodore P. Hipkens

SEVERAL WEEKS ago I attended a conference similar to this one. An old clinician friend presented one of the major papers. He commenced his remarks by decrying and deploring what he called "the current age of the managers." He was, with nostalgia, recalling the days when he could provide high quality, low number service at his own pace and under his own rules.

It is perfectly true that twenty years ago my friend established a very excellent agency, serving a very high-quality menu to a relatively small group of people. It is further true that his agency is still operating in the same vein, though increasingly pressured to broaden its service base. It is also perfectly true that for every person well served by him, there are literally hundreds who could profit from his service, but who are not permitted to by reason of the continuance of the "cottage industry approach" to the distribution of health services.

I tell you this to warn you that I speak to you today from the point of view of the manager—from the point of view of the manager who, given a mission or an assignment, takes time to assess the means available to him; invites the assistance of competent, technical and professional staff advisors; gathers all information possible having a bearing on the mission; formulates tentative, alternate courses of action towards the achievement of his objective; perhaps designates a final objective in broad terms and selects several intermediate objectives that may be accomplished along the way; and finally makes a decision as to how to go about organizing his resources to best achieve his mission. He builds into his final plan a degree of flexibility that permits a quick response to unexpected targets of opportunity that may present themselves along the way; or, similarly for unexpected roadblocks. I would like to discuss factors within this background:

1. The Appalachian Regional Hospital health care system.

2. The utilization of the principles under which rehabilitation facilities have operated for years, their application to the problems of rural health care delivery, and their long experience with true team delivery of services as well as their focus on functioning human beings rather than pathology.

3. How Appalachian Regional Hospital is using certain mechanisms to achieve better distribution of health care in line with the rehabilitation principles.

4. Some general rules that ARH found useful in organizing for optimum delivery of rural health services. Although they are specifically related to ARH, I think that with minor modifications these general rules are applicable to the organization of the delivery of health care in most areas.

THE STORY OF APPALACHIAN REGIONAL HOSPITALS

Appalachian Regional Hospital is only eight years old. In 1956, the chain of 10 hospitals was opened, having been built by the Miners Memorial Hospitals Association, a subsidiary of the Welfare and Retirement Fund of the United Mine Workers of America. If you will visualize a map of central Appalachia, starting in the lower southeast corner of Kentucky at Middlesboro, coming up the ridge line of the Appalachians through Harlan and Whitesburg, over into Virginia at Wise, on up into Kentucky at Williamson, and over into West Virginia at Man and Beckley, each hospital about an hour away from the nearest one, a chain of ten ultra-modern hospitals at that time, in 1956, staffed with full-time salaried physician specialists and prepared to bring modern hospital care and medical care to that area of Appalachia. Financial problems dogged them from the start, and by 1962 the word went out that they were going to be closed or made available for operation by someone else. Through the catalytic efforts of the United Presbyterian Church and aided by the Governor of Kentucky and other interested citizens, a voluntary, nonprofit corporation was formed and named Appalachian Regional Hospitals. It was able to get enough money to buy the hospitals *in toto* from the Miners Memorial Hospital Association and continue them in operation. However, they are now beginning to become community hospitals.

After the first several years and a series of fiscal crises, they began to feel somewhat out of the woods in terms of pure survival and set themselves two major goals for future operations. One goal was to maintain good, traditional community hospitals. More important, however, is the second goal. They committed themselves to using these hospitals as a baseline for the development of all sorts of innovative and imaginative health-related services for the areas they served. Since 1966, these two missions have been uppermost in the planning and execution of the ARH missions.

I said at the outset that I would try to help you understand how Appalachian Regional Hospitals, as they went about trying to achieve their two missions, began to lean heavily on some of the principles long since developed and used by first-class, comprehensive rehabilitation facilities. It was recognized that the concept of team care was a useful one and the rehabilitation facilities could well tell us how to do it. It was recognized that the rehabilitation facilities were aware that there were more components, particularly in dealing with the problems of chronic disease, and that to ignore all these other factors completely often meant wasting time on dealing with the basic physical or medical impairment. We also recognized, however, that we had to convert the terminology and concepts of the rehabilitation facilities into something that was understandable and acceptable to the health care folks.

REHABILITATION PRINCIPLES AND THE CONCEPT OF LEVELS OF CARE

Rehabilitation facilities have developed four common principles, common threads if you wish, that are applicable to the rehabilitation of the severely handicapped. First, of course, there is the requirement that the impairment itself be reduced as far as possible. More important, however, is the recognition that with the severely handicapped one must also work at reducing all of the obstacles to optimum functioning—in other words, work at the total handicap. In addition, conditions and staff attitudes must be fostered to insure that the impairment reduction and total handicap approach has the best chance possible. Such conditions and attitudes can be loosely categorized as a therapeutic climate. Therapeutic climate is an old term. The people in the mental health field have been using it for years, but it is just as applicable to rehabilitation facilities and certainly other health care facilities as well. Finally, the rehabilitation facility people have found that in working with the problems of the severely handicapped (this often can be interpreted as people with multiple "chronic disease and disability") there must be built into the program a mechanism for follow-up in the best sense. It must be continuing and complete.

We have tried to take these rehabilitation facility principles and interpolate them into health care jargon. Admittedly, they are not directly transferable, but under the "levels of care" concept we have found avenues of approach to the utilization of rehabilitation facility principles that are otherwise often difficult to introduce into a traditional general hospital or community health center.

For our purposes we speak of six levels of care: intensive and/or coronary care; intermediate or traditional acute care; extended care; home care; ambulant care; and self-care. We have found it much more possible to introduce these rehabilitation facility principles, for instance, into home care. We expect to find the same applicable in extended care as well as self-care, than, for a lot of reasons, in traditional hospital wards. In pursuing the "levels of care" concept, Appalachian Regional Hospitals has done a number of things.

Under ambulant care, we have begun to build clinic buildings adjacent to our hospitals; we have begun to build satellite clinic buildings away from, but related to our hospitals; we have increasingly brought on full-time, salaried emergency room physicians and technicians; and we are increasingly providing the first contact, the first medical contact, that is, in our emergency rooms. We expect to proliferate our establishment of satellite clinics, which are, in many instances, nurse practitioner managed.

Under the heading of extended care, we have three extended care facilities under construction and two more on the drawing board. We have medical rehabilitation facilities in four of our hospitals already and another on the drawing board. We have vocational rehabilitation facilities in all of our hospitals full-time; we have mental health units in at least five of our hospitals and another on the drawing board.

Foremost in our efforts, the easiest and most seductive level of care to get at has been home care. You will note that I say home care, not just home health, for our home care includes an attempt to get at all of the obstacles to maximal functioning with a given patient, such as nutrition, economics, education, vocation, and social factors. They are even using our pharmacists in a clinical pharmacy sense in our home care teams. We have been willing to ride this horse just as hard as we can, including a willingness to provide satellite home care units in non-ARH communities. However, our focus is constantly on the total handicap of the patient. Home care is ideally suited to the practical application of rehabiltation facility principles. We feel similarly about prospects for extended care.

I indicated earlier that I would discuss primarily our experiences in Appalachian Regional Hospitals, but I also stated there were many general rules developed or discovered which are generally applicable to the organization of health care delivery in rural areas.

GENERAL RULES

There are no pat answers. There are no neat organization charts. The minute you have the one and only way to do it, you have thereafter delimited the opportunity to respond to change and special situations. Each community has its own special collection of characteristics to which the delivery system must make adjustments.

No more hospital beds. That does not mean that old, obsolete beds should not be replaced but, in general, we have the feeling that we have enough hospital beds. We are also convinced that there is at work what I shall call "Hipkens' Law" with regard to new, additional hospital beds. And, "Hipkens' Law" says that if you build a new hospital bed, someone will fill it! Of course, with this generalization goes the implication that in the absence of more hospital beds one must develop other alternate, more appropriate levels of care and this, of course, is what we have been doing.

Proliferate the new services from an established baseline—not necessarily a hospital. It is easier from an existing base for the most part, although I must confess that hospitals tend to be the most monolithic, rigid social structures that one can encounter. Very often in rural areas it may be, however, the only viable social agency available.

Be willing to be an enabler or catalyst or facilitator. Do not feel that the empire has to be all yours. In our case, for instance, we have had several ways of developing physician clinic buildings. In some instances, we have leased land for mental health groups to build mental health clinics adjacent to our hospital. In some instances, we have been willing to provide a wide variety of supportive services to other agencies establishing themselves, ranging from simple purchasing to full management services.

Assign proper organizational status to all levels of care. This means that you cannot organize a home care unit and make it a subgroup of a subgroup within your hospital if you want it to have an appropriate opportunity to grow and prosper and to be a really significant level of care. The same applies to extended care, as well as ambulant care. Each of these levels of care must report directly to no less than an assistant administrator level in a community health center. To make them just one more department of a hospital implies that they really are not very important and will consequently be viewed and utilized as a secondary or tertiary level of care. At ARH an extended care unit, even though physically attached to a hospital building, is a separate organizational entity with its chief manager reporting directly to an assistant or associate administrator.

Ensure equitable rewards to "other" levels of care workers. This means, consistent with the previous general rule, workers in the other levels of care must be appropriately and properly rewarded, including commensurate pay, status, etc. Every effort must be made to point out to both "insiders" and "outsiders" the importance of these other levels of care, so that they are perceived by both the users and the providers as such.

With opposition, look for "soft spots." Invariably, as you try to develop new ways of doing things in old established surroundings, you may expect to encounter opposition, harassment, apathy, etc., and combinations thereof. We have found it very poor tactics to respond with frontal attack as a countermeasure. We have attempted to introduce our new ideas into areas and in fashions that are the least threatening to the status quo, nibbling at the flanks and attempting to surround the opposition rather than overwhelming it directly.

Consider the program manager concept. In this instance, I am talking about a patient program manager. I am saying that in a multi-level community health center it is extremely important that there be provision made for providing easy access for the patient (appropriate access on the part of the patient, continuity, nonduplication, etc.). Particularly, the 15 to 20 per cent of patients with multiple problems need some focal point to manage the patient's total program. Rarely is this properly a physician. More often than not, it may be someone with a background in social work or rehabilitation counseling or any number of health-related professions or subprofessions who can more properly provide this case management function.

Develop an understandable and explainable concept (for staff, trustees, community). This is what we have tried to do in delineating our version of the levels of care concept. The levels of care concept, as we have outlined it here, is readily explainable and understandable. It enables us to convey a useful message to a variety of interested citizens as well as staff.

In all of the foregoing, be guided by the principles of rehabilitation of the handicapped converted to health care terminology. We find that rehabilitation facilities have a great deal to offer from their experience in helping us better organize ourselves to deliver comprehensive health care, particularly in rural communities.

In conclusion a) it is highly desirable that there be active, genuine, collective-cooperative action in organizing for better health care delivery; b) rehabilitation principles converted to levels of care concepts are extremely useful—their concepts of team effort, concern for people, *et al.;* c) Appalachian Regional Hospitals have applied these concepts as outlines; and d) some of the general rules we utilized have usefulness beyond Appalachian Regional Hospitals.

Finally, I turn to Bob Sigmund whose fame as a health care planner is well known. Bob has said that one of the most important aspects of planning involves "asking the right questions." In all our efforts perhaps the key question we inevitably ask ourselves is "What's in it for people?"

CONSUMERS' VIEWS OF HEALTH PROBLEMS

MARTHA ANN CRIDER

My VIEWS are not that of a Doctor of Philosophy or of one who knows or has done extensive study into the questions of why such acute problems exist in the delivery of health care in rural areas. However, I do speak with authority as a low-income person from a rural area and a consumer of health services.

I feel I am fortunate in that I have been on both sides of the health fence. I am on the receiving side as a consumer, and, as president of the Board of Directors of the Mountaineer Family Health Plan, Inc., Raleigh County's Comprehensive Health Project, I have been on the delivery side. I feel fortunate in being on the delivery side, because I have seen and dealt with many problems the average consumer and the general public do not know exist.

I wish to comment first on the receiving side. Rural residents suffer a distinct disadvantage in receiving health care because of the following: a) the geographical situation; b) lack of transportation to urban health clinics and hospitals; c) lack of education of what may be a health problem needing immediate attention; d) lack of funds to purchase health care; and e) lack of information and understanding of state and county operated health programs and agencies.

I am happy to say the Mountaineer Family Health Plan, Inc., a delegate agency of the Raleigh County Community Action Association, has dealt effectively and efficiently in all of these problem areas. The project is unique in that it not only delivers care to the low income community, but the low income community is involved in and plays a major role in the delivery of care through the efforts of community action.

217

Health agencies, like consumers, have their problems. These problems boil down to one thing: not having enough money to implement the care which the program is designed for and has proposed to do.

Health projects must operate within a budget. With the rising costs of medicine and hospital care it is increasingly more difficult to purchase care to operate a comprehensive health project.

Presently, the Mountaineer Family Health Plan, Inc. in Beckley, Raleigh County, has a total of 15,000 persons eligible and receiving care under the Plan. This figure is roughly 22 per cent of the county total, with a possible 10,000 more eligible.

But, of course, the question of funds to take care of the people boils down to what Congress feels are the priority problems in this country. If the Congressmen feel that the war, foreign aid, and supersonic missiles are more important than providing this country's poor with much needed care in order that they may enjoy healthful lives, then, in fifty years, there will be nobody with enough good health to fight a war. It is the boys from poor families that are doing the fighting.

I would like to further air my views of "preventive medicine," the popular term in health circles. You cannot be preventive unless you consider all the causes of the problem; you cannot be preventive unless you have the necessary resources. A rural resident may have so many existing disadvantages that his future health is placed in jeopardy. His water usually comes from a branch or hole beside the road; his water does not have fluoride; he still has his outdoor toilet. In winter his family may have constant colds, because of the dilapidated condition of his home. What can one come up with that is preventive that will solve this problem?

A large percentage of mothers still use "belly bands" for their newborn. Although many doctors say this is unnecessary, the mother will say, "I don't care what the doctor says, I don't want my baby to have a ruptured navel." This is prevention on a small scale. But, if that child has a weak abdominal cavity, nothing short of an operation will correct the abnormality, no matter what she does. What I am saying is, rural families have a weak cavity.

Regardless of the band, unless you go in to correct what is causing the problem, all outside efforts are superficial.

Congress is treating a weak cavity because Congress cannot see the vast need for more appropriations than are presently being provided for health care in this country. Congress must realize the dire need for funds to adequately take care of the low income, elderly, and indigent citizens of this country, especially those who are caught in the squeeze of not being eligible for the OEO and Federal-type program.

Congress is using a belly band. It is not costing much money, not as much as an operation would cost, but the fact remains that an operation is necessary to correct the situation.

I sincerely hope that out of this conference may come some concerted effort toward legislation and the reconciliation of health problems.

CONSUMERS' VIEWS OF HEALTH CARE PROBLEMS

Leonard J. Pnakovich and Eli Zivkovich

T HE CRISIS in health care is one of many in our society today. Without reservation we are convinced that the subject before us is important from a national as well as from a West Virginia point of view.

Fortune magazine in 1970 stated what is wrong—"The biggest obstacle in the path of a more rational medical system is organized medicine."

We claim to be the richest nation in the world, but we have millions living in poverty; in West Virginia 65 per cent of our population suffers and lives in poverty.

We have a surplus of food, yet millions suffer from malnutrition. We are led to believe that American medicine is the best in the world; we are told that we are the healthiest people on earth, but the statistics reveal that we are not.

We have for too long lived with the crisis of health care; deficiencies in health care services and remedies for resolving them were spelled out many years ago, but to no avail. The whole structure and system of health care is antiquated and out-of-date. The more we try to repair it, the more we expose its failures to meet the current needs. Effective change is needed now, for you cannot afford to be sick in America. A comprehensive report in 1932 on the ways and means by which the delivery of health care could be effectively organized suggested health planning with community participation. Nothing has been fully achieved in these past forty years.

Private insurance, whether nonprofit or commercial, has failed to protect the consumer of health care against exploitation and quality defects and has now enslaved him financially.

Blue Cross and other insurance companies have sold the basic policies which force people to get diagnosis and treatment in hospitals where costs are the highest; they have refused to experiment with paying for preventive care and out-patient diagnostic procedures at local community clinics and health centers. The neglect of preventive medicine, the concentration on expensive hospital beds, and the resulting unnecessary surgery and admissions have been the sad and iniquitous contribution of insurance leadership to the present health care crisis. Blue Cross's failure in cost control of hospitals is not surprising.

The health service industry will not be allowed for too long to function in total disregard of public interest and necessity. Look at the major abuses and conflicts of interest which are neither ethical nor professional, i.e. drugs, eye glasses, blood programs, and chain operations of patient beds. A 1971 study revealed that the drug industry spends more than 4,000 dollars per year per practicing physician on promotional activities. The array of cocktail parties, entertainment, color advertisements, and gimmicks, and the gift-bearing salesmen have become a notorious backdrop for an industry which resists the use of generic terms in prescribing drugs which would result in sensible pricing for commonly used drugs and protective controls for patients.

Most physicians do not own a piece of the action at the local pharmacy, but some do. A few more have kickback arrangements which may take the form of expensive gifts or choice tickets to athletic events. A few physicians regard this as improper. Nevertheless, they own shares in repackaging houses which directly siphon profits from the trade name prescriptions the same doctors write. Still more own stock in ethical national pharmaceutical firms for whose products they write prescriptions regularly. It is time to ban this kind of interlocking relationship with suppliers.

Similar connections exist in connection with laboratory work and the ordering and dispensing of eye glasses between ophthalmologists and opticians and the manufacturing companies. The medical society's tactical delays involving physician members with private interests in commercial blood banking are reported to have kept the American Red Cross blood program out of Chicago for four years.

Deserving sharp criticism are nonprofit community hospitals whose inefficiencies are widespread and whose boards of directors are self-perpetuating limited in-groups denying representation to broad sectors of the community.

We must also regard as evil the propriety chains which are now spreading from the skilled nursing home business into the hospital industry. American Medicorp, a Pennsylvania-based outfit, controls thirty hospitals and plans to acquire seven more with a total bed complement of 5,815. Hospital Corporation of America, of Nashville, controls twenty-three hospitals and plans to acquire an additional twenty-seven for a total bed count of 6,715. Extendicare, Inc. of Louisville with fourteen hospitals and a bed count of 1,886 and American Medical Enterprises of Los Angeles with thirteen hospitals and 1,854 beds are representative of the new corporate enterprises. On the major exchanges and in over-the-counter stock markets such companies use local franchises, stock options, and warranty rights to secure viable outlets in local markets. Major stock holdings and corporate leadership are often held by physicians and some companies actually require physician stock participation at the local hospital or nursing home level.

Such profit-making hospitals may eliminate emergency rooms, refrain from taking Medicare or Medicaid cases, deemphasize education, and have not the slightest intention of offering comprehensive health care programs for the community. They run sharp cost-cutting operations.

Physicians ownership in such proprietary or chain institutions is a conflict of interest which contributes to excessive billing, poor quality service, and unnecessary hospitalization.

This country is fast moving toward some kind of national health program which appeals to the middle class who lives in comfort but is otherwise threatened with 100 dollar-a-day hospital charges. And, these charges are moving up the cost graph at an alarming rate. These upward moving health care costs will create a reaction and crisis as they threaten to wipe out savings and the comforts of daily living.

Acceleration of charges and rising premium costs for inadequate health insurance is the number one health problem facing the people today—the black and white, the poor working people, the middle class, and particularly organized labor. Collective bargaining agreements have usually included monetary increases for health benefits, but no more than one-third of the costs has been covered and many essential health services have been omitted.

To meet the escalating costs of health care, organized labor has had to run hard to keep pace, while at the same time its consumer members have become medically sophisticated. The United Mine Workers of America Welfare and Retirement Fund is an example of a unique national program providing one segment (the miners) of the nation's work force with almost total comprehensive medical care of high quality.

IS RURAL UNITED STATES REALLY AN UNDERDEVELOPED COUNTRY?

HELEN L. JOHNSTON

Is RURAL United States really an "underdeveloped country?" This question crossed my mind as I heard Dr. Roemer review the rural health achievements of many countries in Latin America, Asia, and Africa as well as in Europe and North America. Some of these countries have taken massive steps toward improving rural health services and the manner of their delivery. Yet some of these same countries have been the objects of foreign aid and technical assistance from this country. Is it possible that we need some foreign aid and technical assistance in reverse to help us solve our rural health problems?

I also wondered what motivated these countries to place such emphasis on health measures. Is it possible there were sound economic reasons such as a healthy worker is a productive worker, and a healthy country is a productive country?

If so, is there something wrong with our economics and possibly our sense of values? Yesterday we heard a strong argument for developing health services only in viable economic "growth centers." As we compare health indicators such as infant mortality in our country with the rates of some of the other countries mentioned by Dr. Roemer, we find ourselves lagging considerably behind. The question is, can we solve such problems by locating our health services only in growth centers, or do we need to get the services out where the people with the problems live?

As we have talked together, we have focused closely on health. Yet the subject of economics continues to come up, whether in relation to the economic support of health services or in relation to new jobs within or outside the health industry so that people can afford to purchase care. Why do we continually fragment health

224

from other efforts to improve individual family and community living? Are there ways in which we can put our fragmented efforts together and thus serve people more effectively?

Dr. Roemer might have mentioned a rural model of integrated effort that was once tried successfully in this country. Just about a generation ago, the Farm Security Administration was "invented" to help desperately poor rural families all over the United States regain an economic foothold. It started by emphasizing loans to poor farmers who lacked funds even to purchase seed, fertilizer, and other necessary supplies to plant their fields in the spring. These farmers could not qualify for loans from any other source.

After a short time, the Farm Security Administration found that some loans were not being repaid on time. They investigated further and found that in many cases, the meager income of their borrowers was being used to pay medical or hospital bills. There were no funds left to repay the loan. In some cases the premature death of the family head led to failure to repay the loan.

Still further investigation through a sample survey showed a heavy burden of illness and disability among FSA's family borrowers. As a result, the FSA coupled a health program with their economic program. They employed "outreach" workers, called family advisors, who worked with their borrowers and helped them plan use of their resources, including an allowance for the cost of health care as well as the costs of meeting other family needs. County-wide associations were formed and negotiations were conducted with local medical societies for payment for health care in advance on a capitation basis. In some cases it was possible to encourage physicians to set up a small group practice. Consumer participation, group prepayment in advance on a capitation basis, and negotiated arrangements with physicians were all present in these county-wide health plans for Farm Security borrowers.

A quarter of a century ago this beginning of what could have become a nationwide rural health program was terminated by Congress—not because it did not work but because at that time it was too "radical." Now we are calling similar developments "health maintenance organizations" and they are being accepted as conservative rather than radical solutions to existing health problems.

When Mr. Hipkens discussed the Appalachian regional hospital system, I wondered where the element of "participatory democracy" was that we have talked about at other points in this conference? In Dr. Roemer's presentation, also, there was no mention of consumer participation with providers in decision-making regarding health care delivery.

The developments discussed this morning indicate the disparity between the "community of the problem" and "community of the solution." In the case of the Appalachian regional hospital system, each community might have looked at its own problem and considered itself the "community of the solution" as well as of the problem. But, in this case the real solution was not in a single community but in a linkage of one community with a number of others. Otherwise in some cases local health services could not have survived. Shared effort by a number of communities on an organized basis not only gave each one additional security; it also enabled them to offer a level of care beyond what any one of them could have maintained alone.

In the foreign countries, also, the community of the solution was not the single rural community but rather the nation as a whole.

We seem to be moving in this direction. Recent legislation has been enacted by the Congress which can have special value to rural areas of West Virginia, Appalachia, and other parts of the country. The Coal Mine Safety Act is, of course, pertinent only to areas where coal is mined. Most of these areas are rural. A friend recently called my attention to the fact that the Act includes a requirement that mine operators provide or assure the availability of emergency health services to miners and their families. As yet there is no specific legal interpretation of this requirement. Citizens of the coal mining towns of this area should be seeking support from the United Mine Workers, their health and welfare agencies, and comprehensive health planning bodies to assure a broad interpretation and full implementation.

Another recent piece of legislation passed by the National Congress is the Emergency Health Personnel Act. This has promise for helping to meet critical health manpower shortages in "medically underserved" areas of the country—rural and urban. The majority of the examples of need cited during Congressional hearings were from rural areas. Rural people of West Virginia were represented in the hearing by Dr. Nolan. Other rural areas were represented by similar professional and lay leaders.

Dr. Leslie Dunbar commented that he believes we are on the verge of major welfare legislation, legislation that may set the pattern of welfare service delivery for a generation. Similarly, we are on the verge of major health legislation—milestone legislation not unlike the Hill-Burton Act of twenty-five years ago. When the Hill-Burton Act was being considered, the voices of rural people and their organizations were heard in Congress. As a result, provisions were built into the Act for meeting the special needs of rural areas. During the generation since the Hill-Burton Act was passed, hundreds of small community hospitals have been built. They now dot the landscape of rural America.

Now rural people have another chance. As the voices of the Mrs. Criders, the Mrs. Browns, and the Dr. Nolans from West Virginia and all the Nation's rural areas are heard, the future of rural health in this Nation will become brighter.

THE FAMILY HEALTH SERVICE

ROBERT EAKIN

D<small>R.</small> R<small>OEMER</small> has reviewed critical dimensions of rural health services in international perspective, and has thereby given us a broad view of how rural health services might be organized. I shall discuss the dimensions identified by Dr. Roemer and comment on Mr. Hipkens presentation in terms of our experience in a particular comprehensive health project and its institutional context in a rural, mountainous area of north-central West Virginia. The project I refer to is the Family Health Service, a division of the Memorial General Hospital Association, Inc., in Elkins, West Virginia, where I serve as Administrator. This project, which is funded primarily by a grant under Section 314 (e) of the Public Health Service Act, is designed to bring approximately 20,000 disadvantaged rural people into the mainstream of comprehensive health services by eliminating the barriers of ignorance, timidity, lack of transportation, and lack of adequate financial resources. We were fortunate in being able to start with a well-developed set of medical services and facilities including a multispecialty group practice composed of 22 physicians and dentists, a 151-bed general hospital, and a 105 bed convalescent hospital providing extended care and long-term care. To these elements we added the Family Health Service providing outreach and social services, home health care, home nursing service, home environmental services, health transportation and Family Health Fund.

PREVENTION OF DISEASE

The home environmental health program of the Family Health Service is directed toward the control of unhealthful environmental factors that may affect individuals living in a particular household. Examples of this type of environmental threat to personal health are insect and rodent infestation, unsanitary methods of waste disposal, dilapidated and overcrowded housing, and polluted drinking water. The ultimate objective is to improve the health of the people served through preventive measures designed to eliminate causes of disease. Another objective is to reduce recurrences of the same illness and thus reduce readmissions, etc.

GETTING THE DOCTOR TO RURAL AREAS

It is apparent to us that a physician will be more likely to go into a rural area where there is a well-developed health care system. Also, it has been our experience that a group practice can attract physicians to a rural area because of advantages it offers in professional relationship and financial security. In addition, the financial support provided by the Family Health Fund gives encouragement for a physician to come to a low income rural area, since he can reasonably expect to receive payment for his services.

ANCILLARY HEALTH MANPOWER

We have trained twenty-three indigenous women as Family Health Workers. Recruited from the small communities located throughout the county, they serve in a dual role as a health advocate and home health aide. Among their many tasks they serve as an outreach worker, a casefinder, and a referral agent for all social agencies, as well as promoter of health programs in their communities.

RURAL HOSPITALS AND HEALTH CENTERS

The Memorial General Hospital and the Golden Clinic recorded in excess of 118,000 out-patient visits last year. During the same period ambulatory care increased 18.1 per cent, while in-patient admissions rose only 9.2 per cent and total patient days decreased 3.8 per cent. In our judgment the decrease was, in part, due to the Family Health Service programs including home evaluation, nutrition, home health care, health transportation, and financial assistance for timely medical treatment. A group practice located within the hospital permits the hospital to function extremely well as a health center. The combination of these health care components permits more efficient and convenient utilization of the diagnostic and treatment facilities and a resulting reduction of overhead and administrative costs. The "economy of scales" recognized in the manufacturing industry is prevailing. The shared services concept related by Mr. Hipkens is a good example and should serve to moderate the rate of increases in costs.

TRANSPORTATION AND COMMUNICATION

Two health vans transport patients to health care providers by traveling regularly scheduled routes. Experience has proven that the vans are used almost entirely by those who are completely indigent and who reside primarily off the main and more heavily populated routes. A regularly scheduled health transportation system permits many patients to participate in programs which are directed toward preventive and health maintenance who might otherwise not have the opportunity to do so.

A radio communication system has been funded for use by the Family Health Workers, nurses, social workers, and health van drivers. In addition to emergency use, we will be able to maintain closer supervision, to provide more timely instruction and direction, and to increase health services. We expect to reduce travel and other costs. Consequently, a more effective service will be rendered to the residents in all aspects of outreach and home health care programs. An added advantage is that the Family Health workers' feelings of isolation will be greatly reduced.

ECONOMIC SUPPORT

A Family Health Fund is operated to assist families to pay for health services based on the family's annual income and size. As can be expected, a disproportionate amount of funds are expended for care of families in the lowest income categories. Nearly 6,400 families have registered or participation in the program. We have estimated that approximately 8,800 families are eligible to participate in the Family Health Fund. The need for financial aid in paying for health care for rural people is evidenced by the following statements. The vast majority of registrants (71 per cent) are in the low income levels and qualify for 70 per cent or more financial assistance. The fund is operated on a last dollar concept. The Family Health Fund is paying 72.5 per cent of the health costs for their members, while the family and third party pay the balance. The acceptance of the program by the people has been excellent. Nearly all the health providers in the community are participating in the program. Those few who are not participating support the program in principle.

HEALTH PLANNING AND COORDINATION

The Memorial General Hospital Association has endeavored to establish a health delivery system which provides for care of the patient at the most appropriate level as determined by his physician. Mr. Hipkens' statements on this concept strongly support our approach. Although elimination of rising hospital costs is not possible in this time of increasing wages, however, it is reasonable to anticipate containment of costs to individual patients treated at the most appropriate level of care. I must emphasize, however, the urgent need for adequate financing for programs of all levels of care, including extended, long-term, and custodial services. Cooperation of many health providers has been achieved with a major degree of success in the operation of the Family Health Service. Strong support has been received from the consumers (i.e. those registered for benefits with the Family Health Service) and others. Collective action, referred to by Mr. Hipkens, existed throughout the development of the project and continues today. Planning and coordination is necessary in the health care delivery system, and, in my opinion, has been paramount in the success that the programs of the Family Health Service have achieved to date.

EXPERIENCE OF TWO FAMILY
HEALTH WORKERS

Garnett Bentley and Doris Haddix

We both come from small communities in Randolph County, West Virginia. Helvetia and Pickens both have under two hundred residents. We live about thirty-five to forty miles from the nearest doctor.

Our work as family health workers for the Family Health Service of Elkins consists of two main parts: home health aide and outreach worker. As home health aides we are assigned patients through the nursing department of the Family Health Service following a doctor's referral and orders. We go into the home of the patient with the nurse when she makes her first evaluation visit, and following that, we carry out her and the doctor's orders. Examples of this type of work are medication checks, catheter or colostomy care, and decubitus ulcer care. We are trained also in first-aid to help in emergencies.

As an outreach worker we function in four different ways: a) as a good neighbor; b) as a health advocate; c) as a social service aide; and d) as a community organizer.

As a good neighbor we go into the homes for case finding when a new family moves in or on the occasions of birth and death. We explain the Family Health Service to them and at the same time learn about the needs of the family. We also tell them about the services available to them, for example, the twelve-passenger van that comes out into our areas once a week to take people into the health providers of their choice. When in the home of a newborn, we check to see that clothing, food, and the other necessities for proper care are in the home. We also ask about the health of the other family members, such as immunizations for the other children in the home.

232

Second, as a health advocate we encourage people to avail themselves of the medical resources available as health problems arise. This includes encouraging general good health habits for keeping well, such as getting people started on a regular physical and dental examination schedule. For example, we have a woman living in our area who had not been to a doctor for over ten years. We checked her blood pressure and it was extremely high. After two or three visits to her home we finally convinced her that she should see a doctor. However, she lived up in a hollow and never traveled to town. When the van was in our area, one of us went with her for her first visit to the hospital and to see a doctor. Now, we are happy to report, she goes on her own and she goes regularly.

Third, as a social service aide we refer people through the Family Health Service social worker to other service agencies such as the Food Stamp Program, Vocational Rehabilitation, Crippled Children's Service, and other resources available in Randolph County. For example, we have a man in our community who is fifty-one years old with a wife and eight children. At the age of 13 his arm had been amputated. Through a referral from our office, this man will soon be fitted with an artificial limb. Specific patient assignments may be made by the social worker to work with families who have a health related, environmental, social, or emotional problem.

Fourth, as a community organizer we help to set up community health programs as necessitated by health needs. For example, we helped to organize forums for the White House Conference on Aging. We also organized classes for the first aiders, attendants, and drivers for a satellite station of the Randolph County Emergency Squad. Because it takes about an hour and a half for an ambulance to come from Elkins to our area, in January of 1970, we worked with the ambulance squad in Elkins to form a satellite station in Pickens. We have made many successful runs and we operate with only volunteers. Also, community organization includes helping to publicize other agencies' programs such as health department clinics for immunization, pap smear, or chest x-ray and family planning clinics.

Most significantly, the people recognize us in our communities. They accept us because we are a neighbor. We know the language and the customs, and the people know that we are just a phone call away. Even though we are part-time workers, we are usually on the job twenty-four hours a day.

HEALTH EDUCATION ADVISORY TEAM

BARBARA JONES AND JOAN WHITE

THE HEALTH Education Advisory Team is a nonprofit, consumer health organization which receives its funds through a grant from the United States Department of Health, Education, and Welfare Public Health Service.

It was created in June, 1969, in response to the need to bridge the communication gap between the medical providers and medical consumers. A staff of Health Advocates was hired to go into the communities to find what the health needs are and if the consumers are taking advantage of the existing programs.

The founders of HEAT determined that the providers were not sufficiently informed about the health needs of the citizens of Marion County, especially those consumers in the low income areas. HEAT set out to rectify this situation through a program designed to educate consumers as to their rights to quality health care services.

By making consumers aware of their health needs, HEAT was able to organize an effective, persuasive consumer health organization which sought to bring about the necessary changes needed to upgrade the medical services provided by Marion County; to encourage the coordination of health services with consumers and providers at the local, state, and regional levels; and to encourage the use of new and innovative approaches to the delivery of health services in Marion County.

THE COMMUNITY AND HEALTH CARE

The crisis in the delivery of health care necessitates inputs from many sources. Traditionally, responsibility for the development of health services rested with the providers of medical care.

Recently, members of communities across the country have

become involved in the health care system on a new level. They are sitting on boards and working with organizations in newly defined roles as health consumers. Under federal legislation they are sharing in the responsibility for policy formulation and planning of future health services.

The Community Health Corporation was designed to meet the needs which have emerged as the community participates in decision making in the health field.

It is the mission of HEAT to provide an improved health care delivery system to all consumers in Marion County, especially those in the lower income bracket, and to ensure that these consumers are aware of the benefits available to them through the HEAT program.

The objectives of HEAT are as follows:

1. To promote a positive partnership between the health consumer and the health provider.

2. To provide consumer groups with the tools for effective participation.

3. To cooperate with health institutions in developing a constructive working relationship with consumers.

4. To sensitize the broader community to health problems and stimulate involvement in the search for solutions.

NOTES ON ENDING THE CONFERENCE
GAP

ROBB BURLAGE

HEALTH conferences often lack sufficient representation of either the "consumers" in whose interest real solutions now are life and death matters or the "controllers" of the established resources; these must be fully reorganized and redistributed if real solutions are to be forthcoming. Where is the opportunity to conspire publicly among those interested in solutions and where is the opportunity to confront publicly those who must be moved?

In Appalachia there is the peculiar dichotomy between a reputation for new health projects in the framework of persevering health problems. Here are some of the most celebrated rural health projects launched in previous decades (e.g. coal miners hospitals, medical groups, and frontier nursing). Appalachia is also known for some of the most visible federal rural health project appropriations, occupational health activities, and compensation legislation of this decade (100 million dollars-plus for Appalachian Regional Commission "health demonstration areas," plus the Coal Mine Health and Safety Act, including disabled coal miners and widows black lung compensation).

Despite this, Appalachia has deeply enduring, escalating crises involving rural medical, industrial, and environmental survival in the 1970's. Are its tarnished projects, severe problems, and social and environmental imbalances atypical or merely melodramas of the essential national situation?

What does "rural" mean in this part of the industrial heartland, so close to vast natural wealth, and in this immediate area close to considerable health institutional resources? Conditions in nearby Preston County, West Virginia shocked our own senior United States Senator when he toured health problem areas with

Senator Kennedy recently. Yet, it is only a few miles from the state's major medical center. Although it is a rural area, is it not socially similar to an industrial slum only minutes across New York City's East River from four medical school "empires," and, like our rural areas, essentially unattended by ambulances and with no health services? Are we talking about "pockets" of poverty and exceptionally remote, depressed areas where some areas experience overwhelming problems involving transportation, accessibility, and industrial dislocation? Or, are we talking about the very heart of the American political and economic anatomy?

We observe a nation increasingly "urban" in available services, socially integrated, with secure mobility for the rich, but increasingly socially remote and rural with insecure migration for the working poor. We see a politically oriented economy of high energy use and complex technology yielding national "macro-growth" but deadly to the lungs, lives, livelihood, and land of a socially "rural" majority, whether "inner city," "gray area," "small town," or "extra-urban."

During the late 1960's, obfuscating words about new federal health programs float down to us: comprehensive health planning, medical center regionalization, health maintenance organizations, applied biomedical research, and national health insurance. Are we waiting in line for trickle-down federal projects or new federal policy, instead of working to reconstruct the control and direction of health services where we are?

In the very "catchment area" of this conference, in the shadow of West Virginia's major medical center, which is also heartland Appalachia's only medical school, it must be reported that there has been more done by major medical administrators to obstruct and to divert new reconstructive energies in the health area than anything else. For example, some University Medical Center, local medical society, and local, general hospital representatives, among others, have failed in a number of attempts to obtain federal funding for a new county nursing home facility. They were told this was at least partly because there had been no comprehensive health planning in the county. They then convinced county officials to spend public funds on an architectural consulting firm to do a "health planning survey" for the county. The painfully predictable results: no real involvement of consumers in the survey, even in interviews. Also, there was no real consideration given to decentralization, preventive medicine, mental health, or environmental problems, health needs, or alternative approaches. There was no analysis made of health financing needs and alternatives or of means to make health services publicly accountable and provide for "system integration." The total emphasis of the survey was on a proposal for a private foundation, a coalition of University Medical Center, general hospital, and medical society representatives to build a private super-hospital, nursing home, and medical office building complex, presumably to be designed by the same architectural firm. There was no discussion of the feasibility of such a new central hospital complex, although the survey proposed to reprieve the University Medical Center from its responsibility as a public institution for the discrimination, negligence, and disorganization with which it now provides emergency, chronic, and general care. The survey describes it as a state educational institution with no immediate community health responsibilities.

A group of health consumers in the county is now challenging this provider planning process and its sadly limited results. As part of the county and regional comprehensive health planning process, they are carefully creating citizen public hearings, including close cross-examination of major health providers and representatives in the county (including the University Medical Center) to determine their activities and plans. They intend to stimulate consideration of local system alternatives, such as an elected county health authority, a network of community health centers, and a comprehensive program of prepayment for health services for all citizens. Some of these same active citizens of Monongalia-Preston County areas next door to the state's major medical center have been further shocked to discover that in this supposedly most enlightened medical area we are surrounded by two major group practice programs (represented in the program of this conference) in adjacent counties but none in this county. Further, a major union-community prepayment program is being organized in Western Pennsylvania on our northern border, although no such efforts have been mentioned by our own Medical Center leadership.

An additional example of established obstruction in our area has affected the efforts of local rural citizens. In communities with great medical need, they have tried to organize community health centers with their own doctors and with the help of some University Medical Center house staff, medical students, and paramedics in an attempt to serve such areas, at least on a volunteer basis. Despite departmental support, such proposals have been constantly rejected and even threatened. In one community, people are, nevertheless, going ahead on their own to create a community free clinic, obtaining their own malpractice insurance, equipment, and drugs. The same medical administrators who deny support and obstruct the efforts to develop health services claim the key problem in rural health is the lack of awareness or diligence of the people themselves. Let us note that the public is becoming increasingly aware of where the central problem is, where the desperately needed resources are, who has the power now, how the consumer public might gain more leverage, and what must be done to move in these directions.

It is ironic that despite the existence of a major federal environmental-occupational laboratory and research center attached to the University Medical Center, there is contemporary obstruction of efforts to improve occupational, industrial, and environmental health. At least an estimated 270,000 miners and widows have been denied federal benefits for black lung disease, with this geographic area experiencing one of the highest denial rates. Rather than taking the lead in major advocacy for hundreds of thousands of coal miners victimized by black lung disease, some spokesmen in these same institutions have made public statements shamelessly and unscientifically slurring the evidence, blandly minimizing the existence and causes of the illness, pointing to cigarette smoking and air pollution (anything but the coal companies) as the cause.

The University Medical Center has had a number of grave lead poisoning cases, almost all clearly related to work at a particularly local metal processing plant. In a manner which suspiciously tends to favor company management, the Medical Center has failed even to advise patients of the full significance of this disease, let alone their compensation rights, the true industrial cause, and supportive measures to achieve prevention and early detection. However, employee groups, miners, disabled miners and widows, steelworkers, and others in this area have begun seeking their own direct professional advice and have been taking their own action regarding compensation, prevention, and alternative health plans. This also includes University and Medical Center employees, who themselves face serious occupational hazards. As employees they were given notice that they would lose access to the University Health Service. Only when the employee groups vigorously protested was that plan revoked.

I have mentioned these few local "cases" not only to challenge the present systematic obstruction within established medical system resources, but also to emphasize the new seeds of health system reconstruction provided by the consumers. I also wish to acknowledge the people with seemingly obstructive institutions, including those who called this conference, who are making yeoman efforts to make breakthroughs with new services, and to acknowledge that these institutional actors in such cases apparently see their own definitions of public responsibility in a different way. We should take note from these "victims" of rural health care who are beginning to take and demand action and are obtaining increasing assistance from front-line health workers. Let us try to get together beyond pleasant gatherings that listen to systems management summarizers, project reporters, and rambling theses of potential legal fiat. Let us begin to talk directly to each other about what we are really doing and must do in practice in our particular areas against the sometimes curiously evasive responses of the medical system. Let us summarize all the possible themes in one chorus and one word: NOW!

INDEX